AF800428

Ketogenic Diets

Treatments for Epilepsy and Other Disorders

Eric H. Kossoff, MD
John M. Freeman, MD
Zahava Turner, RD, CSP, LDN
James E. Rubenstein, MD

16
EasyRead Large

RHYW

Copyright Page from the Original Book

Acquisitions Editor: Noreen Henson

Cover Design: Steven Pisano

Compositor: Apex CoVantage

Printer: Bang Printing

ISBN: 978-1-936303-10-6
E-ISBN: 9781617050640

Visit our website at www.demoshealth.com

Medical information provided by Demos Health, in the absence of a visit with a healthcare professional, must be considered as an educational service only. This book is not designed to replace a physician's independent judgment about the appropriateness or risks of a procedure or therapy for a given patient. Our purpose is to provide you with information that will help you make your own healthcare decisions.

The information and opinions provided here are believed to be accurate and sound, based on the best judgment available to the authors, editors, and publisher, but readers who fail to consult appropriate health authorities assume the risk of any injuries. The publisher is not responsible for errors or omissions. The editors and publisher welcome any reader to report to the publisher any discrepancies or inaccuracies noticed.

Library of Congress Cataloging-in-Publication Data

CIP data is on file at the Library of Congress.

Special Sales Department
Demos Medical Publishing
11 W. 42nd Street
New York, NY 10036
Phone: 800-532-8663 or 212-683-0072
Fax: 212-941-7842
E-mail: rsantana@demosmedpub.com

Made in the United States of America

11 12 13 14 15 5 4 3 2 1

Set in 16 pt. Verdana

Important Note to Readers

This book introduces the ketogenic diet to physicians, dietitians, and parents of children with difficult-to-control seizures who might benefit from the treatment. This book is not intended to be an instruction manual. A book cannot take into account the specific needs of any individual patient. As with any course of treatment for epilepsy, a decision to try the ketogenic diet must be the result of a dialogue between the parents and their child's physician.

THIS DIET SHOULD *ONLY* BE INITIATED under the supervision of a physician and a trained dietitian or nurse.

If you are reading this book, we assume that you are familiar with the basic descriptions of epilepsy and what they mean. This is not a book about seizures or epilepsy. This is about one form of treatment for epilepsy—the ketogenic diet.

This book is dedicated to the memory of Ms. Diana Pillas

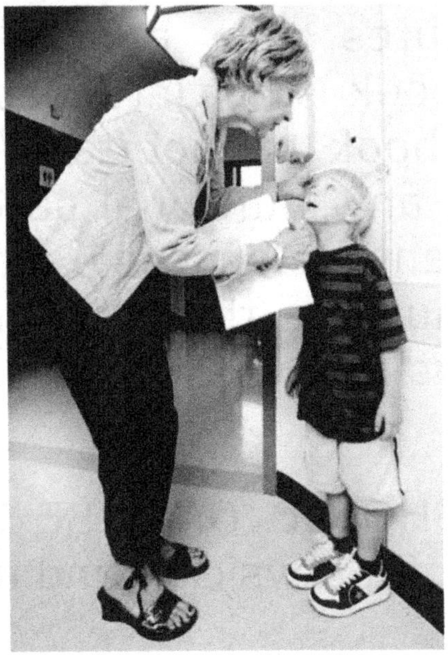

Courtesy of Mr. Keith Weller, photographer.

Diana was the face of the John M. Freeman Pediatric Epilepsy Center for three decades until her unfortunate death due to breast cancer in February 2010. She was the heart and soul of our center, providing advice, support, and a shoulder to cry on for countless parents and children.

She was the primary source of information for those families specifically considering dietary therapy, and based on many factors, she would even sometimes discourage some families from the diet. For these families, she would often suggest a treatment that would be more likely to succeed. Other times, she would fight with insurance companies and usually encourage me to squeeze in a child she knew in her heart would do great on the diet.

There was nothing we loved more than seeing Diana smile and nod knowingly when we told her a child she helped put on the diet was seizure-free. We'd like to think somewhere she is reading this book and smiling—many of her creative ideas led to research projects, which then made the diet easier and more effective for children around the world. Her incredible insight, wisdom, and love for children are sorely missed.

Foreword

On March 11, 1993, I was pushing my 1-year-old son, Charlie, in a swing when his head twitched and he threw his right arm in the air. The whole event was so subtle that I didn't even think to mention it to my wife, Nancy, until a couple days later when it recurred. She said she had seen similar incidents. That was the beginning of an agony I am without words to describe.

Nine months later, after thousands of seizures, an incredible array of drugs, dozens of blood draws, eight hospitalizations, a mountain of EEGs, MRIs, CAT scans, and PET scans, one fruitless brain surgery, five pediatric neurologists in three cities, two homeopaths, one faith healer, and countless prayers, Charlie's epilepsy was unchecked, his development "delayed," and he had a prognosis of continued seizures and "progressive retardation."

Then, in December 1993, we learned about the ketogenic diet and the success that Dr. John Freeman, Millicent Kelly, RD, and Diana Pillas had been having with it at Johns Hopkins Hospital as a treatment for children with difficult-to-control epilepsy. We took Charlie to Johns Hopkins. He started the diet. Charlie was seizure- and drug-free within a month. Today, he is a happy, healthy, 18-year-old high school senior. He eats whatever he wants, has no recollection of his epilepsy, and has very little memory of his 5 years of diet therapy.

Back in 1994, when we realized that a vast majority of Charlie's seizures and most of his $100,000 of medical, surgical, and drug treatments were unnecessary—even harmful—we founded The Charlie Foundation To Help Cure Pediatric Epilepsy in order to help promote and increase the diet's usage. Among other efforts, we supported the first edition of *The Epilepsy Diet Treatment.*

Today, though the mechanisms of diet therapy remain the same, the diet itself has grown in accessibility, palatability, understanding, and popularity almost as much as the now 6'1" Charlie has grown in height. Due in large measure to the earlier editions of this book, many of the myths that impeded my family, and so many others, from awareness and access to diet treatment have been dispelled—leading to a ground swell of patient and parent knowledge and empowerment. Most importantly, this has led to thousands of healthier children.

It is our continued hope that *Ketogenic Diets—Treatments for Epilepsy and Other Disorders—Fifth Edition* will help others decide whether the diet is a viable alternative to their current treatment.

And we know this book will be an invaluable guide once diet therapy has begun.

Jim Abrahams, Director
The Charlie Foundation to Help Cure Pediatric Epilepsy

Preface

Back in the dark ages of the ketogenic diet during the 1980s, the response to a diet that was 90% fat was, "Yuck!" Everyone—physicians, the public, and parents—all *knew* that such a high fat diet was unpalatable, unhealthy, and couldn't possibly be a treatment for anything. Fat was thought to be bad, and the ingestion of such a diet would inevitably lead to heart disease, strokes, and death. "A diet for treating epilepsy? Crazy, we're still trying to find the proper medication(s). We're not looking for unsubstantiated alternative therapy." "All that's true is rarely new, and all that's new is rarely true."

Over the ensuing decade, the high fat, ketogenic diet has been shown to be palatable, not unhealthy, and highly effective in treating many forms of epilepsy, and perhaps other diseases as well. Indeed, it is more effective and less toxic than any of the current anticonvulsant medications.

The concept of a mere diet being able to control otherwise uncontrollable seizures seemed far-fetched to many back in 1994, when we reintroduced the ketogenic diet with the initial publication of *The Epilepsy Diet Treatment: An Introduction to the Ketogenic Diet.* Seventeen years later, with the help of the first four editions, the ketogenic diet has become a widely accepted therapy for children with difficult-to-control seizures. It has won over skeptics and gained acceptance among both physicians and the public. Medical centers around the world are developing the expertise needed to administer the treatment successfully. The limiting factor in its use seems to be the lack of adequately trained dietitians who are the prime ingredient in the diet's implementation and success.

There are few new therapies in modern medicine that have come to the fore in so short a time. Modern medicine still treats most epilepsy in children and adults with anticonvulsant medications. Because it is based on food, the ketogenic diet is considered by many to be an *alternative therapy.* However, it is one of the few alternative therapies that has, through careful controlled studies, shown demonstrated success and become a part of mainstream medical treatment. We, therefore, no longer consider it *alternative.*

Since the first edition of this book was published, and even since the most recent fourth edition, a *huge* amount of new information has been generated on the ketogenic diet. This is the reason we felt a new edition was needed. Two landmark randomized, controlled trials have shown the world that the diet works. Recent and ongoing studies suggest that the former rigidity of the standard ketogenic diet may not always be needed, and we believe this new edition reflects the *relaxing* of the rules a bit. This is especially true in the last 10 years, during which the *alternative* ketogenic diets have been actively used—the modified Atkins diet and low-glycemic index treatment (LGIT); an entire section devoted to these treatments is now included in this edition. The title of this book is no longer *THE Ketogenic Diet,* but *Ketogenic Diets!* The diet is being used more and more for adults and even for conditions other than epilepsy.

More countries than ever are using the diet in sometimes innovative ways. The ketogenic diet is not just the "Hopkins diet." This edition, unlike any other before, has contributions from dietitians at several other centers who will share their keys to success.

Although once thought to be the treatment of last resort, used only when all medications have failed and when surgery for the epilepsy was not an option, the diet is now considered when a child has failed only one or two medications and may be a treatment of initial choice for infantile spasms. This idea, hopefully a sign of things to come, is the subject of an entirely new chapter in this edition.

The diet has come a very long way, and this fifth edition book marks another milestone along its path. But even today, with all the new anticonvulsant medications that come on the market, there are still many children and adults with difficult-to-control seizures. The ketogenic diet, if properly done, remains more effective than any of these new anticonvulsant medications. It seems clear that if the diet were a drug, companies would be heavily promoting it as the treatment of choice for difficult-to-control epilepsy. We have been fortunate to have the support of several companies that make ketogenic formulas and supplements, but even that support is limited.

CAUTION: The ketogenic diet should *ONLY* be used under close medical supervision. The decision to use the diet should be the result of a dialogue between physicians and parents. It is rarely successful without the continuing support of an experienced physician and a knowledgeable dietitian.

The ketogenic diet is NOT the answer for everyone's seizures. But even so, it may be worth trying. The diet is more effective than any of the anticonvulsants on the market after medications have failed and with fewer side effects. More than one-half of the children with difficult-to-control epilepsy who attempt the diet achieve more than a 50% control of their seizures, which is nearly twice the average (about 30% who respond to a new drug). Dr. Helen Cross showed that nicely in her study from 2008. They are usually able to reduce or eliminate their antiepileptic medications and may remain seizure-free even when the diet is discontinued. For many, it may result in a better quality of life with fewer side effects than any other current therapy.

There still remain many, many questions about the ketogenic diet. We do not yet understand fully how it works, but *that* it works is clearly established. This new edition of *Ketogenic Diets* reflects the many advances in understanding that have taken place since interest in the diet was resurrected and the first edition of this book published 17 years ago.

Eric H. Kossoff, MD
John M. Freeman, MD
Zahava Turner, RD, CSP, LDN
James E. Rubenstein, MD

Acknowledgments

The authors would like to express our appreciation for the invaluable help we received from the many contributing authors and reviewers of this book. As demonstrated by their work on this edition, the world of the ketogenic diet is growing rapidly. We would like to thank the following individuals:

- Dr. Mackenzie Cervenka
- Dr. Adam Hartman
- Jim Abrahams
- Beth Zupec-Kania, RD
- Elizabeth Neal, RD, PhD
- Heidi Pfeifer, RD
- Bobbie Henry, RD
- Millicent Kelly, RD
- Susie Gingrich, RD
- Jennifer Bosarge, RD
- Chef Neil Pallister-Bosomworth
- Gerry and Michael Harris
- Michael Koski

SECTION I

Overview of the Traditional Ketogenic Diet

CHAPTER ONE

Epilepsy Today and the Place of the Ketogenic Diet in the World

WHAT IS A SEIZURE ANYWAY?

Many families who come to see us at Johns Hopkins have not been even told what epilepsy is. *Epilepsy,* other than being a scary word, just means more than one seizure. There are many children with epilepsy who are at the top of their class in math and science, and several more in colleges on varsity sports teams. However, other children are not so fortunate.

Epilepsy is not a very useful word for our affected families unless it helps them put a name to their child's condition, a condition that in some cases does not have a clear answer. There are many causes of epilepsy, so the name itself is not often helpful, except to get services or explain it to family members and neighbors. This is very frustrating, needless to say. The good news is that for situations when neurologists can't say definitively why a child is having seizures, they also can't say definitively if a child won't outgrow the seizures either. Sometimes no news is good news.

After a single seizure, we often (not always) obtain an electroencephalogram (EEG). In general, there is a 30% chance of a second seizure. On the other hand, there's a 70% chance that the child will never need to visit us (other than for social reasons) ever again due to being seizure free. It is for this reason that most neurologists do not start medications after just one seizure except in very unusual circumstances.

Once a second seizure occurs, the risk flips, with a 70% chance of a third seizure. When this seizure will happen isn't clear, although typically children with abnormal EEGs are even more likely to seize sooner rather than later. Unless the two seizures are very far apart in time, we will often start medications to try and prevent more seizures.

MEDICATIONS

All the available medications are meant to help, not to cure. Only time (and a little prayer) will lead to a cure for many of the children we care for. When seizures are impacting a child's quality of life, medications are not just a good idea, they are important. Twenty years ago, we only had a handful of medications. In 2011, we have more than 20 medications—double that of two decades ago.

Many of the newer medications have a kinder side-effect profile, although relatively few are approved by the FDA for children, especially those under the age of 2 years. Neurologists will choose a drug depending upon the cause of the seizures and the seizure type. Drugs can be "first-generation," such as Tegretol® and Depakote®, or "second-generation," such as Trileptal®, Keppra®, and Topamax®. More and more frequently today, we are using the newer drugs earlier and in some cases even first.

Despite all these new medicines, it is not clear to us that the child with difficult-to-control epilepsy is much better off. The children that did not respond to medicines in the past are not responding now. In about two-thirds of children, the first drug used is successful without side effects. If side effects occur, there are new drugs available to take its place right away. Those children might respond to the second or third drug.

Sadly, about 10% don't respond to any drug. Many recent studies in both children and adults have shown that if two or three drugs don't work, stop wasting your time with a fourth or fifth drug and move onto other options. This is typically where the ketogenic diet is used.

WHAT ABOUT WHEN MEDICATIONS FAIL?

Even after one drug has failed, most neurologists nowadays think about whether brain surgery is an option. In some cases, it is. Those children, although certainly facing some risk in the operating room, have a very good chance (especially if there is something clear on the MRI, PET, or MEG scan) of having their seizures cured by surgery. However, there are even more children who are not clear candidates for surgery, as listed in Table 1.1.

TABLE 1.1 Why Surgery Would Not Be an Option

- Many different regions of the brain where the seizures originate
- Seizures coming from an important area of the brain (movement, language, or memory)
- Too risky for some children with other medical issues
- Source of seizures not clearly found despite EEG with electrodes placed on the brain
- Some are generalized seizures (e.g., petit mal or Lennox Gastaut)
- Bleeding disorder
- Not able or willing to travel to a center that does surgery regularly
- Family (and child) not willing to take the risk

When surgery is not an option and medications fail, children are left with few options. These mostly include dietary treatments and vagus nerve stimulation (VNS). Depending upon who the doctor is, one of these therapies is typically recommended. At our hospital, as you would expect, we recommend the diet first almost always. Other hospitals, often those with less experience with diets or more familiar and comfortable with VNS, will recommend the diet only after a VNS is unsuccessful.

Our experience, similar to most centers, is that a VNS is often a help but rarely a cure, and probably less commonly a cure than the ketogenic diet. The diet usually works quickly (studies suggest often within the first month of use), whereas VNS often takes months to work. The VNS is generally without side effects (hoarse voice, cough, possible infection), other than the risk of general anesthesia required for the brief surgery. Most of our patients have had some improvement, but also seem more alert and interactive. We are very interested in the combination of both the ketogenic diet and VNS at the same time as using both together sometimes seems to work better than each alone (in limited research). We tend to rarely use a VNS in children under the age of 3 years.

WHERE DO DIETARY TREATMENTS FIT IN THIS PLAN?

This is where the ketogenic and modified Atkins diets, as well as the low-glycemic index treatment, are commonly used. We have seen some dramatic results with diets for even the toughest of seizure cases. The diet is continuing to grow in use both in the United States and worldwide. Much of this success is a result of the work of the Charlie Foundation, a parent support group that has championed the use of dietary treatments in the United States since the mid 1990s (www.charliefoundation.org). Further information about this wonderful group and other groups around the world is in Chapter 13. The diet can be given to young infants, teenagers, and adults. Side effects are generally few and often reversible should they occur without having to stop the diet.

WHAT ABOUT OUTSIDE THE UNITED STATES?

In the 1990s, as the ketogenic diet was starting to grow in popularity in the United States, other countries were also beginning to use this treatment as well; notable countries include England, Germany, Australia, and Canada. Since that time, there has been a virtual explosion of interest all over the world. In 2011, over 50 countries offer the ketogenic diet, with many countries having multiple centers to choose from! We still receive emails from parents in Europe and Asia stating that the ketogenic diet is "not available" in their country and they'd like to come to Baltimore, but this is rarely necessary today. Each country is more familiar with its own cultures and foods, so we usually refer these parents to appropriate ketogenic diet centers. A list of these centers is provided in Appendix D and at www.epilepsy.com/ketonews.

However, there are still barriers to widespread use of diets around the world. Many regions of the world do not have ketogenic diet centers, especially Central America, Southeast Asia, and Africa. Some of this is poverty related, but there is also some unfamiliarity with dietary treatments as well. Work is underway in Honduras, India, and China to bring the modified Atkins diet (which may be possible to undertake with limited dietitian support and cost) to these regions.

Also, some parts of the world do have ketogenic diet programs but have long waiting lists due to their particular health care systems. This is more difficult to navigate around, but we usually advise parents to be proactive for their child, keeping in frequent contact with their neurologist, and trying to be moved up the waiting list if seizures start to worsen.

TABLE 1.2

Outcomes of the Ketogenic Diet: Johns Hopkins Patients, 1998

Number Initiating	Seizure Control and Diet Status	Time After Starting the Diet		
		3 Months	6 Months	12 Months
Total: *N*=5150	100% seizure free	4 (3%)	5 (3%)	11 (7%)
	> 90%	46 (31%)	43 (29%)	30 (20%)
	50–90%	39 (26%)	29 (19%)	34 (23%)
	< 50%	36 (24%)	29 (19%)	8 (5%)
	Continued on diet	125 (83%)	106 (71%)	83 (55%)
	Discontinued diet	25 (17%)	44 (29%)	67 (45%)

Source: From Freeman et al., Pediatrics 11/98.

DOES IT WORK?

Multiple studies have shown that slightly more than half the children on the ketogenic diet will have half of their seizures improve (Table 1.2). About one-third will have a >90% improvement. About 10–15% will be seizure-free, and when this occurs, everyone is thrilled. Studies show that the diet is particularly effective for conditions such as infantile spasms, myoclonic-astatic epilepsy (Doose syndrome), Rett syndrome, Glut-1 deficiency, tuberous sclerosis complex, and children receiving formula only (such as through gastrostomy tubes or an infant bottle).

Megan,[1] a highly motivated 12-year-old with a supportive family, was able to "cure" her seizures after 2 years on the diet. Here is a letter written by Megan's parents after she had been on the diet for just 6 weeks.

MEGAN'S STORY

DEAR DR. FREEMAN,

I want to share with you and your team the wonderful changes in Megan's life since she has been on the ketogenic diet.

As you remember, we were having very serious and frightening prospects as a family....

---

1 Some names in this book have been changed to protect the privacy of the patients.

Megan's seizures, which we called "stares," were out of control in spite of using three drugs. She was experiencing so many an hour that she was regressing both in school and in her personal skills. She would be unable to remember what she had been doing prior to a "stare," and therefore had difficulty staying focused on tasks—whether keeping her place in her reader or even dressing herself, or just remembering what she went to get in another room.... Being only 10 years old, she was very frightened because she was not able to stop "staring," and children teased her. She cried because she would wake up at night and not realize she was in her own bedroom. She also described many auras in which she reported seeing flashing lights and people's faces changing colors...

We could not increase the Depakote ® level because of the side effects to her stomach. She was taking Mylanta three times daily just to coat her stomach to tolerate the Depakote ®. And still her stomach hurt, resulting in poor appetite—which ... had reduced her weight to the tenth percentile for her age group. This constant concern over her eating patterns and small consumption had also created tension in our family over meals.

The ... seizures also resulted in her ... sleeping at least 12 to 13 hours out of each 24, including sleeping an hour at school midday.

As a result of all these physical changes, the disorder now took Megan's social life. Since she had to go to bed so early, she couldn't go to church or ... school functions. On Saturdays, she could play only in the morning because she would sleep in the afternoon. Spending the night with a friend became out of the question because she didn't get enough sleep—which increased the "stares." Her neurologist recommended Johns Hopkins Hospital and your team because he felt surgery would have to be considered—that Megan would likely become worse.... And so we came, expecting to have to chance even losing her life in order to give her the chance of improving quality of life—and save the very essence of our spirited, enthusiastic, loving child.

Due to the complexity of Megan's neurological situation, you did not recommend surgery, but offered her something incredible—a diet! You told Megan she could use her strength to turn down sugar from her friends and to stay on her diet. We will never forget how her little face lit up when you said "no surgery."

Her life has literally turned around from that day.... She has been very dedicated to learning about labels with sugar, preparing foods, etc., and is determined to stay on her diet.

It has been and will be worth the extra time it requires to plan and prepare the meal plans. She has had only two "stares"—one the day of dismissal from the hospital, the other at school when she began decreasing the Dilantin level.

She has really had a learning spurt. Her reading teacher ... tested Megan and ... confirmed the improvement in reading already! Megan is thrilled to be promoted to a harder reader. Her memory also improved, and she is being assigned more difficult words. She is choosing her clothes and dressing herself with little supervision from me. She is going to slumber parties!

Family and friends say over and over they can tell how well she is doing. Her thoughts are well connected in conversation. Megan says, "I'm so much better than before I went to Baltimore. I can remember things now. I'm doing great!" In short, she is alert and happy.

After seven and a half years of dealing with frequent and frustrating medication changes with varying side effects, this diet is a fantastic alternative. I will not complain! This Christmas was our most joyous since the first Christmas after she was born.

The diet was not easy. Megan's family had to learn step by step how to organize life around the diet for 2 whole years. Megan cried the time she won a spelling bee in her class and the prize was a pizza, of which she could take not even a single bite. "I shared it with all of the class, but I couldn't have any myself," she later recalled. Megan's own motivation, as well as her supportive family, were important keys to making the diet a success. The fact that the diet was 100% successful was highly motivating and its own reward.

Megan remained on the diet for 2 years and has now been off the diet for 12 years—seizure-free and medicine-free. Despite structural damage to her brain from the epilepsy and a mild hemiparesis, she has just graduated from high school and plans to go on to more studies. Asked if the diet was worth it, Megan replied, "It gave me my life back."

Megan's story is dramatic, but many similar letters have been written by grateful parents. Articles about children with 100% success stories have appeared in newspapers and periodicals around the country, with headlines such as "Michael's Magical Diet," "Cured by Butter, Mayo and Cream," "Epilepsy's Big Fat Miracle", and "High Fat and Seizure Free." These are the glowing reports of the dramatic success that the diet can achieve.

The diet is not as difficult as it used to be years ago. Ketogenic formulas (e.g., KetoCal®) can be used as baking mixes to make foods that normally contain flour. We are not as strict as we used to be about calories, fluids, and the ratio. This is a big difference in this edition of *Ketogenic Diets* compared to the 4th edition. KetoCalculator (Chapter 9) has made more recipes than ever available to families. The modified Atkins diet and low-glycemic index treatment are also available for those few who can't tolerate the ketogenic diet (and also for teens and adults);

more on this in Section IV. You and your child *can* do it.

DEFINING SUCCESS

Unfortunately, the ketogenic diet does not result in a success story for everyone. Almost half of all children who start the diet stop during the first year. Some stop because, despite the medical and support team's best efforts to "fine-tune" the diet, and despite the family's diligent efforts, the seizures have not improved sufficiently to make their efforts worthwhile. Some discontinue because of illness, noncompliance, or because the diet is "just too hard."

> *For example, Jay was a 15-year-old whose seizures started at age 9. In the 6th grade he had so many dizzy spells and seizures that he missed 77 days of school. In the 7th grade he was taking 16 pills per day and still missed 108 days of school. He had brain surgery in which his temporal lobe was resected, but the seizures returned. Jay and his family then decided to try the modified Atkins diet.*
>
> *Jay's goal, like that of many teenagers, was to be able to drive. For this he needed to be 100% seizure free. On the diet he fell short of this goal—he was nearly seizure free, but not completely. Five months after starting the diet, Jay's mother reported that he "lives on sausages, eggs and choked-down heavy cream at every meal." "We are always in the kitchen ... cutting,*

cleaning, measuring," his parents wrote. "We never go out to eat anymore or have pizza at home.... At Thanksgiving the whole family ate eggs."

Jay's seizures were much improved and his medications were reduced, but without being seizure free, Jay believed that he would never be able to drive and therefore the diet was too much trouble. The diet was discontinued after about 9 months.

With so much improvement in seizure control, was Jay's experience with the diet a success? Well, yes and no. His seizures were markedly decreased and his medications were reduced. However, his major reason for undertaking the diet was to become 100% seizure free so that he could drive. Because he wasn't able to reach this goal, the diet was—for him—a failure. This is sometimes a problem for adults who we start on the modified Atkins diet.

Similarly, we have had children in whom the number of seizures is unchanged, but the parents strongly believe it is helping. The seizures might be shorter, less intense, or occurring only at night, for example. Some children are able to reduce medications and are more alert, despite the seizures not slowing down. Even though the total numbers of seizures may be discouraging to our ketogenic diet team, the parents may believe it's a success and want to stick with it. Ultimately, it is the child and the parents who must define the diet's success or failure.

WHEN SHOULD THE DIET BE USED, THEN?

Most experts believe diets should be considered after two or three medications have been tried. If a child's seizures are well-controlled with medications and experiences no side effects, the diet is not necessary. Children with infantile spasms and Doose syndrome may be exceptions to this rule, and we have used the diet first in those situations with excellent results. Details are in Chapter 24.

However, for some, even with seizures under fairly good control, medication may affect children's alertness and mental clarity, impairing their ability to learn and reach their full potential. Therapy for epilepsy is often a balance between seizure control and medication toxicity.

The point at which an individual's seizures are deemed out of control, or side effects are considered unacceptable, varies from person to person and from family to family. Most children who start dietary treatment are having at least weekly (and usually many per day) seizures. In a study of parent letters written at the time the diet was started, we found that most mothers and fathers agreed and wanted seizures and medications reduced. Most were realistic and didn't expect seizure or medication freedom. Surprisingly, 9 out of every 10 parents requested something else: typically improved alertness, less injury, or improved performance in school.

Following are actual excerpts from a note from a 23-year-old currently on the diet for the past 10 years.

> *Before I started the diet, I was having seizures constantly! I would also get dizzy spells from the medications I was taking at the time. About 6 months into the diet, my family and I started seeing a change in my behavior. I was more alert, more understanding of my surroundings, and able to use my fine motor skills at a faster pace. I remember the first month that I did not have any seizures at all! I was 14 and I was jumping up and down inside! When it came time to total up the amount of [seizure] activity for that month, I drew a big fat zero and made it into a smiley face.*
>
> *It has been 9.5 years since I started the diet. I am now 23 years old and am on a 4:1 ratio. One of the things I like best about the ketogenic diet is that I get to pick what I want to eat from a variety of menus which coincide with the diet's restrictions. Out of all the menus I have to choose from, I enjoy cheese and broccoli soup during the winter, as well as omelets; I also enjoy peanut butter and bacon, as well as egg salad during the summer.*

One hundred seizures a day is clearly too many, but are three seizures a month too many? Some children and families consider that limiting seizures to one a week a victory, while others consider one seizure every 2 months an intolerable state of affairs. Varying degrees of sedation, hyperactivity, and learning disabilities may be acceptable in exchange for seizure control. But what if you could control seizures without such side effects?

This is a question asked by many parents. Could my child learn better, faster, more easily without the toxicity of the medication? Would her behavior and attention improve if she weren't on anticonvulsants? How can you tell when a child cannot be taken off medication without the chance of recurrent seizures?

The net result is that many children and their parents look beyond currently available medications for a satisfying solution to seizure treatment. For many parents, the ketogenic diet, which does not have the same level of cognitive and behavioral side effects of many anticonvulsant medications (especially older ones such as phenobarbital), offers a chance—sometimes an unattainable dream—of seeing their child free of medications and seizures. For many parents, it is as important to see their child free of medication as to see them free of seizures. For others, like Jay's family, described previously, the ketogenic diet is not considered a success because the seizures were not completely eliminated. Even in those who discontinue the diet, however, most find the attempt at the diet worthwhile because, as they often say, "at least we know that we tried."

The ketogenic diet simulates the metabolism of a fasting body. A fasting person burns stored body fat for energy; a person on the ketogenic diet derives energy principally by burning the fat in the diet rather than from the more common energy source, carbohydrate (glucose). As the water content of a fasting body is lower than normal, so the ketogenic diet limits liquid intake and lowers the water content of the body. But unlike fasting, the ketogenic diet allows a person to maintain this fatburning, partially dehydrated metabolism over an extended period of time.

> *We fought for the diet against our doctor's advice. My son's seizures were fairly well controlled; he was only having maybe one a month or every six weeks. He was having them more often before we started the latest medication a few months ago. He was on three drugs at high doses. However, he was cranky and moody all the time. His doctor said, "This kid's seizures are pretty much under control on the medicine. What more do you want?" What I wanted was for my boy to get his old, sweet personality back.*
>
> *He has had seizures only when he is sick now and is down to a low dose of just one medication. He likes himself now and other kids like him. We*

> *hope to eventually stop the diet and hopefully his seizures will stay under good control.*

Success on the ketogenic diet requires the commitment, determination, and faith of the entire family. Thirty grams cream, 12 grams meat, 18 grams butter—the recipe begins to sound like old witches concocting a magic brew. There is mystery to it. No one understands all the reasons how or why the ketogenic diet works. But it *does* work, and it has worked for more than 90 years.

CHAPTER TWO

What Is the Ketogenic Diet?

The ketogenic diet is a medical treatment for controlling seizures by switching a body's primary metabolism to a fat-based energy source rather than utilizing glucose. The body obtains energy from three major food sources:

1. *Carbohydrates:* Starches, sugars, breads, cereal grains, fruits, and vegetables
2. *Fats:* Butter, margxarine, oil, and mayonnaise
3. *Proteins:* Meat, fish, poultry, cheese, eggs, and milk

Carbohydrates comprise approximately 50% to 60% of the average American's daily caloric intake. The body converts these carbohydrates to glucose, which is burned by the body to produce energy. When the supply of glucose is limited, as during fasting, the body burns its fat for energy. During prolonged starvation, if there is insufficient fat, then muscle is burned, thus compromising energy and good health.

The body maintains only about a 24–36 hour supply of glucose, and once that glucose is depleted, the body automatically draws on its backup energy source—stored body fat. This is a survival skill, inherited from our hunter-gatherer forefathers who may have had to go for prolonged periods between game kills and, during those times, used their stored fat as their energy source.

The ketogenic diet was designed to simulate the metabolism of this fasting. When a fasting person has burned up all his glucose stores, he then begins to burn stored body fat for energy. After the initial fasting period, a person on the ketogenic diet derives his energy principally by burning the exogenous dietary fat rather than from the more common energy source, carbohydrate (glucose), or from their own body fat. But unlike fasting, by providing exogenous fat the ketogenic diet allows a person to maintain this fat-burning metabolism as its primary source of energy (instead of glucose) over an extended period of time.

In the absence of glucose, the fat is not burned completely but leaves a residue of *soot* or *ash* in the form of ketone bodies, and these ketone bodies build up in the blood. The ketone residues are *beta-hydroxybutyric acid* and *acetoacetic acid.* The beta-hydroxybutyric acid can be metabolized by the liver and by the brain as a source of energy. The acetoacetic acid is excreted in the urine and the breath and imparts a sweet smell to the breath that has been likened to pineapple.

When ketone levels are large enough, as indicated by a simple urine test, it is said that the body is *ketotic* (pronounced key-tah´-tic) or in a state of *ketosis.* Ketosis is also evidenced, as mentioned previously, by a fruity, sweet odor to the breath. In the presence of large levels of ketone bodies, seizures are frequently controlled.

THE BASICS

REMINDER: The traditional ketogenic diet is a rigid, mathematically calculated, doctor-supervised therapy. This diet should only be attempted under close medical and dietary supervision.

The ketogenic diet simulates the metabolism of a fasting individual. A fasting person burns stored body fat for energy; a person on the ketogenic diet derives energy principally from the fat in the diet rather than from the more common energy source, carbohydrate. But unlike fasting, the ketogenic diet allows a person to maintain this fat-burning over an extended period of time. Traditionally, the diet has been initiated over 3 days after a 48-hour period of fasting (a limited amount of carbohydrate-free fluids are allowed during this period). More recent studies (discussed in Chapter 7) have questioned whether fasting, slow initiation, or even the traditional ketogenic diet itself is necessary for seizure control.

Foods

Common, but carefully selected, ingredients are used in meals that a child can eat while on the ketogenic diet (see Chapters 8 and 9). With the help of a dietitian and careful calculations, the diet can be adapted to many foods and many cultures around the world (see Chapter 6).

The diet can also be started as a liquid formula for bottle-fed infants and children with a gastrostomy feeding tube. For the parents of these children, the diet can be fairly easy to administer because compliance is not an issue, and the formula tastes as good as regular baby formula.

Can my child live a normal life while on this diet?

The answer is clearly YES! Here are examples of what some ketogenic meals might look like:

Sample meal plans

Breakfast 1
Scrambled egg with butter
Diluted cream
Orange juice

Breakfast 2
Bacon
Scrambled eggs with butter
Melon slices
Vanilla cream shake

Lunch 1
Spaghetti squash with butter
and Parmesan cheese
Lettuce leaf with mayonnaise
Orange diet soda mixed with whipped cream

Lunch 2
Tuna with mayonnaise
Celery and cucumber sticks
Sugarless Jell-O with whipped cream

Dinner 1
Hot dog slices with ketchap
Asparagus with butter
Chopped lettuce with mayonnaise
Vanilla cream Popsicle

Dinner 2
Broiled chicken breast
Chopped lettuce with mayonnaise
Cinnamon apple slice with butter topped with vanilla ice cream

Alternatively, breakfast might include a mushroom omelet, bacon, and a cream shake, or another special Keto-recipe cold cereal. Keto cereal was invented by the creative mother of a child who missed eating his bowl of cereal in the morning. The mother crumbled keto cookies in a bowl and poured cream over them.

This made an excellent cold cereal that satisfied her son. Each meal will depend upon the desires of the child and the imagination of the parent.

> REMEMBER: The ketogenic diet should only be initiated under medical and dietary supervision!

MYTHS AND MISUNDERSTANDINGS ABOUT THE DIET

Contrary to the beliefs of some parents, the ketogenic diet is not "all natural," "holistic," "organic," or "pure." The ketogenic diet is a means of treating seizures in children, and perhaps in adults as well. The diet may be more effective for some forms of seizures than our current medications. It definitely is a substantial intrusion on a family's life. Some families have made it more of an intrusion than others. Some have fed the child on the diet separately from the rest of the family thinking the KetoKid might feel deprived if they saw other food that they cannot have. We feel that this is never a good idea. Rather, one can make the child feel special by emphasizing that he (or she) has a special diet. However, physicians and families must always weigh the difficulties and benefits of the ketogenic diet compared to medications and their side effects and to seizures, and try to do the best thing for each child.

THE DIET is not the best choice for everyone.

The ketogenic diet is not completely free of side effects. In general, the ketogenic diet is better tolerated than most medications and has fewer potential side effects. However, it does have side effects. The major side effects seen with the diet are lack of weight gain, *slightly* decreased growth, *somewhat* high cholesterol, constipation, kidney stones, and acidosis. All are treatable and reversible without having to stop the diet.

Emma, who had epilepsy, is one example. Emma's family thought any diet would be better than giving their daughter drugs. They believed that medications were unnatural and had side effects, so they tried to keep Emma off anticonvulsants. They had tried gingko and St. John's wort and had made several trips to chiropractors and hyperbaric oxygen treatment centers. Nothing had helped her seizures. After a long discussion about the ketogenic diet with neurologists at Hopkins, however, Emma's parents began to recognize that although the diet was perhaps an option, medicines, if effective, would be much simpler! An anticonvulsant medication was started, and Emma became seizure free after 3 weeks. She never had to go on the ketogenic diet.

Charlie Abrahams is an alternative example. For over a year and a half, his physicians had tried multiple medications and even surgery before the ketogenic diet was attempted. His seizures were completely controlled within 1 week on the diet.

The ketogenic diet requires a lot of commitment and a lot of work initially. Medications are easier if they are effective and without substantial side effects. Even for families who become expert in preparing the diet and organizing their lives around it, the ketogenic diet is a big undertaking. Anticonvulsant medications are far easier to use, and if they work, they are probably a better choice than the diet. This is why physicians usually recommend that an individual with seizures should try one or two medications before turning to the diet.

A modified Atkins diet (discussed in Chapter 18) is somewhat easier than the traditional ketogenic diet, but it is still not easy.

Common misunderstandings about the diet

- "The diet will completely control the seizures."

  Some children (about 1 in 10) do become seizure free. Others will have a reduced number of seizures. Half of children who try the diet do not receive enough benefit to make it worth continuing. In any event, the diet is worth trying. If it is too difficult or provides inadequate control, you can always stop the diet (see Chapter 16) and return to trying medications.

- "She will get rid of all those poison medicines that have side effects and are not even approved for use in children."

  This is a result to be desired, but it is not a reality for everyone. First, a child has to have good control of the seizures. Only then the doctor can try to decrease or eliminate medicines.

- "We will just try it for a few weeks, and if it doesn't work we'll go back to medications."

  We ask each family for a 3-month commitment. After starting the diet, it takes 3 months to fine-tune it, which involves finding the correct amounts of calories, finding the correct spacing of the meals, and getting both the child and the parent accustomed to this new lifestyle. Initiating the ketogenic diet requires too many changes and commitments on the family's part, and too much commitment from the whole keto team, to have someone not give it a proper chance.

CHAPTER THREE

History of the Ketogenic Diet

Fasting and prayer have been mentioned as treatments for seizures and epilepsy since biblical times and are mentioned again in the literature of the Middle Ages. However, it was only in 1921 in the journal *Medical Record* that fasting as a treatment for epilepsy was reawakened. At the American Medical Association meeting that year, Dr. Rawle Geyelin, a prominent New York pediatrician, reported the successful treatment of severe epilepsy by fasting.

Geyelin cited the case of a "child of a friend" age 10 years, who "for 4 years had had grand mal and petit mal attacks which had become practically continuous." At Battle Creek, Michigan, he came under the care of an osteopathic physician (Dr. Hugh Conklin), who promptly fasted him, the first fast being one of 15 days. Several subsequent periods of feeding, then fasting, occurred. "After the second day of fasting," Geyelin reported, "the epileptic attacks ceased, and he had no attacks in the ensuing year." Geyelin reported seeing two other patients, also treated by Dr. Conklin, who, after fasting, had been seizure free for 2 and 3 years. He further reported that he had fasted 26 of his own patients with epilepsy, 18 of whom showed marked improvement and 2 remained seizure-free for more than 1 year.

Dr. Geyelin stated that the best length of fasting was 20 days. This was the first U.S. report of the benefits of fasting on epilepsy.

> IT IS OF HISTORICAL INTEREST that the father of Hugh Conklin's patient, "HLH," reported by Geyelin, was Charles Howland, a wealthy New York corporate lawyer and the brother of Dr. John Howland, Professor of Pediatrics at the Johns Hopkins Hospital and director of the newly opened Harriet Lane Home for Invalid Children at Johns Hopkins in Baltimore. In 1919, Charles Howland gave his brother $5,000 to find a scientific basis for the success of the starvation treatment in his son. These funds were used to create the first U.S. laboratories to study fluid and electrolyte balances in fasting children. Although these studies shed light on fluid and electrolyte balance in children and were the start of the investigational careers of many great pediatric physicians, Howland and his team were unsuccessful in finding how starvation helped to control seizures.

The following year (1922), Dr. Conklin published his belief that epilepsy was caused by intoxication of the brain by toxins coming from the Peyer's patches of the intestine. He had developed his "fasting treatment" program in order to put the patient's intestine at complete rest. He stated, "I deprive the patient of all food, giving nothing but water over as long a period of time as he is physically able to stand it ... Some will fast for 25 days and come to the office one or more times every day for (osteopathic) treatment."

WE NOW KNOW that epilepsy has nothing to do with the Peyer's patches of the intestine, but we have learned that fasting seems to curtail seizures.

Dr. William Lennox, considered by many to be the father of U.S. pediatric epilepsy, writes of Conklin's fasting treatment as the origin of the ketogenic diet. Lennox, who later reviewed Geyelin's records, reports long-term freedom from seizures occurred in 15 of 79 of Geyelin's fasted children (18%).

During the early 1920s, phenobarbital and bromides were the only antiseizure medications available. Reports that fasting could cure seizures were therefore exciting and promised new hope for children with epilepsy. These reports set off a flurry of clinical and research activity at many centers.

THE KETOGENIC DIET AND DIABETIC KETOACIDOSIS

Simultaneous with the finding of the effects of fasting on epilepsy, the early 1920s was an era during which early investigations were made into the metabolic basis for diabetes and the often-fatal ketoacidosis that accompanied diabetes. A 1921 review article about diabetes and its dietary management stated "acetone, acetic acid, and ß-hydroxy-butyric acid appear ... in a normal subject (caused) by starvation, or a diet containing too low a proportion of carbohydrate and too high a proportion of fat. [Ketoacidosis] appears to be the immediate result of the oxidation of certain fatty acids in the absence of a sufficient proportion of 'oxidizing' (dissociated) glucose."

In diabetic ketoacidosis, the inability to burn glucose leads to exceedingly high levels of blood glucose, with resulting dehydration of the tissues and chemical imbalances that lead the patient to coma and sometimes to death. These effects clearly do not occur with either starvation or the ketogenic diet, in which glucose is restricted.

THE DISCOVERY OF THE KETOGENIC DIET

Prolonged periods of starvation to hopefully control epilepsy were unpleasant. The first article suggesting that a diet high in fat and low in carbohydrate might simulate the metabolic effects of starvation and its effects on epilepsy was published in 1921. Dr. Wilder from the Mayo Clinic, its author, proposed that "the benefits of fasting could be ... obtained if ketonemia was produced by other means.... Ketone bodies are formed from fat and protein whenever a disproportion exists between the amount of fatty acid and the amount of sugar." "It is possible," Wilder wrote, "to provoke ketogenesis by feeding diets which are rich in fats and low in carbohydrates. It is proposed to try the effects of such diets on a series of epileptics."

The calculation of such a diet, and the effectiveness of Wilder's proposed *ketogenic* diet, was reported by Dr. Peterman from the Mayo Clinic in 1924. Peterman's diet used 1 gram of protein per kilogram of body weight in children (less in adults) and restricted the patient's intake of carbohydrates to 10 to 15 grams per day; the remainder of the calories were ingested as fat. The individual's caloric requirement was calculated based on the basal metabolic rate plus 50%. This is virtually identical to the standard ketogenic diet used today.

Of the first 17 patients treated by Peterman with this new diet, 10 (59%) became seizure free, 9 on the diet alone. Four others (23%) had marked improvement, two were lost to follow-up, and one discontinued the diet. The following year, Peterman reported 37 patients treated over a period of 2.5 years: 19 (51%) were seizure free, and 13 (35%) were markedly improved. These initial reports were rapidly followed by others from many centers. The currently used standard protocol for calculating and initiating the ketogenic diet was well discussed in a book by Talbot in 1927.

Reports of the effectiveness of the diet appeared throughout the late 1920s and 1930s. In these reports, subjects varied and patients were followed up for varying lengths of time. As shown in Table 3.1, early reports of the diet showed 60–75% of children generally had a greater than 50% decrease in their seizures, 30–40% of these had a greater than 90% percent decrease in the seizure frequency, and 20–30% had little or no seizure control.

TABLE 3.1

Reports from the Literature on Seizure Control Using the Ketogenic Diet

			Seizure Control		
Author	Year	Number of Patients	>90%	>50%	<50%
Peterman	1925	36	51%	35%	23%
Helmholz	1927	91	31%	23%	46%
Wilkens	1937	30	24%	21%	50%
Livingston	1954	300	43%	34%	22%
Kinsman	1992	58	29%	38%	33%
Huttenlocher (MCT)	1971	12	—	50%	50%
Trauner (MCT)	1985	17	29%	29%	12%
Sills et al. (MCT)	1986	50	24%	20%	26%

Note. MCT=medium chain triglyceride diet. Source: Representative studies.

The ketogenic diet was widely used throughout the 1930s. In fact, the diet was widely used for conditions such as absence (petit mal) epilepsy, which has recently been rediscovered as a type of seizure that responds well to the diet. It was also used in adults. After the discovery of diphenylhydantoin (Dilantin®) in 1937, attention of physicians and investigators turned from studies of the mechanisms of action and efficacy of the diet toward finding and evaluating new anticonvulsant medications. The new era of pharmacologic treatment for epilepsy had begun. When compared with the promise of the medications, the diet was thought to be relatively difficult, rigid, and expensive.

As new anticonvulsant medications became available, the diet was used less frequently. As fewer children were placed on the ketogenic diet, fewer dietitians were trained in its rigors and nuances. Therefore, the diets prescribed were often less precise, less ketogenic, and less effective than they had been in previous years.

In an effort to make the ketogenic diet more palatable and less rigid, a form of the diet was developed using medium-chain triglyceride (MCT) oil (more about this in Chapter 20). This oil was more ketogenic and allowed for larger portions of food, but children on the MCT diet often suffered from nausea, diarrhea, and bloating; therefore, despite the decrease in seizures, parents often found the side effects unacceptable and gave up. The MCT diet has been recently revised by Neal and colleagues in the United Kingdom to lower the amount of MCT oil and has shown fewer side effects as a result.

Experiences such as these led to the widespread opinion that dietary treatment for epilepsy was cumbersome and difficult to tolerate. Many physicians also erroneously believed that parents and children would not be strong or rigorous enough to comply with the diet. Medicines, and the promise of even more effective medicines on the horizon, were further disincentives to using the ketogenic diet.

THE START OF THE MODERN ERA AND RENEWED INTEREST IN THE DIET

The ketogenic diet continued to be used 6–8 times per year at Hopkins, under Dr. Samuel Livingston and his dietitian, Millie Kelly. Its use was mentioned in our papers on treating difficult seizure problems. Other centers in the United States used it as well, but not very frequently.

In 1993, Charlie Abrahams, age 2, developed multiple myoclonic seizures, generalized tonic seizures, and tonic-clonic seizures that were refractory to many medications. As his father, Jim Abrahams, wrote in the initial foreword to this book, "thousands of seizures and countless medications later," when physicians were unable to help, he began to search for answers on his own and found reference to the ketogenic diet and to our hospital. Charlie was brought to Johns Hopkins, and within 1 week of starting on the diet, Charlie's seizures were completely controlled, his EEG returned to normal, his development resumed, and he no longer suffered the side effects of medication.

Charlie's father wanted to know why no one had told him about the diet before. He found references to the high success rates discussed previously and determined that this information should be readily available so that other parents could become aware of the ketogenic diet.

Creating the Charlie Foundation, Charlie's father, a filmmaker, used his talents to expand awareness and the use of the ketogenic diet. He funded the initial publication of this book. Charlie's story was covered in national magazines and on national television, starting with the news magazine show *Dateline,* further raising awareness of the diet. After the *Dateline* program about Charlie aired in 1994, the 1,500 copies of the first printing of this book were immediately sold out.

When we told him that Johns Hopkins could not conceivably handle the number of patients who would want the diet after the *Dateline* show aired, Jim and the Charlie Foundation funded five pediatric epilepsy centers to allow them to come to Johns Hopkins for a meeting to plan a joint protocol to reevaluate the efficacy of the diet in children failing modern medications. Over the next few years, the Charlie Foundation also underwrote conferences to train physicians and dietitians from medical centers nationwide. Many more medical centers began to use the diet.

Jim created the made-for-TV film *First Do No Harm,* starring Meryl Streep, dramatizing the ketogenic diet. He also filmed our educational efforts about the diet for parents, dietitians, and physicians. He produced videos about the diet for parents, families, children, and for physicians, and he made the tapes available to those audiences. Meanwhile, Nancy Abrahams spent tireless hours coaching and helping other parents during their difficult times with the diet. She spoke at countless parent meetings and conferences, and she provided support for those in need.

After Charlie remained seizure-free for 2 years, he was allowed to come off the diet, but several months later he had a few further seizures. He resumed the diet in January 1996, and he again became seizure-free on a modified form of the ketogenic diet. Charlie has now been seizure-free, medication-free, and off the diet for years. He spoke at the 2008 Phoenix ketogenic diet and is a funny, happy adult.

Without Jim and Nancy's persistence and their dedication to making knowledge of the diet available to other parents, to physicians, and to the public, there is no doubt the ketogenic diet would likely not have been rediscovered so dramatically and would certainly not have received the resurgence in popularity it now enjoys. Considering that most centers around the world started their ketogenic diet centers shortly after the 1998 study funded by the Charlie Foundation, the influence of the Foundation is undoubtedly global.

THE EVIDENCE

The outcome of the initial multicenter funded by the Charlie Foundation in 1998 is shown in Table 3.2. Fifty-one children who averaged 230 seizures per month before starting the diet were enrolled. The study documented that almost half (45%) remained on the diet for 1 year (a measure used in trials of medication to assess both effectiveness and tolerability) and almost half of those (43%) remaining on the diet were virtually seizure-free. Of those remaining on the diet for 1year, 83% had better than a 50% decrease in their seizures.

TABLE 1.2

Outcomes of the Ketogenic Diet: Johns Hopkins Patients, 1998

Number Initiating	Seizure Control and Diet Status	Time After Starting the Diet 3 Months	6 Months	12 Months
Total: N=5150	100% seizure free	4 (3%)	5 (3%)	11 (7%)
	> 90%	46 (31%)	43 (29%)	30 (20%)
	50–90%	39 (26%)	29 (19%)	34 (23%)
	< 50%	36 (24%)	29 (19%)	8 (5%)
	Continued on diet	125 (83%)	106 (71%)	83 (55%)
	Discontinued diet	25 (17%)	44 (29%)	67 (45%)

Source: Reproduced with permission from Vining, Freeman et al. Arch Neurology 1998; 5:1433-1437.

This multicenter study also shows the difficulties of comparing new studies with older ones, which used a different approach to reporting their outcomes. If you look at this same multicenter study from a different angle and include all of those children that the centers "intended to treat," meaning everyone who was started on the diet even if they only remained on it for a day or a week, then, as is shown in the 3rd and 4th columns in Table 3.2, the same 45% of the children remained on the diet for 12 months. But only 10 (20%) of those starting on the diet had better than 90% seizure control at 1 year, and an additional 9 children (18%) had a 50–90% decrease in seizures.

These newer "intention to treat" approaches to reporting clinical trials of treatment give a better concept of the chance of a treatment being effective. If we "intend to treat" a child with the ketogenic diet, the chances of decreasing that child's seizures by more than 90% percent are one in four, according to this methodology.

Since that study, we have started more than 500 children on the diet at Johns Hopkins. Before starting the diet, these children averaged more than 600 seizures per month and had been on an average of more than 6 medications.

As Table 3.3 shows, even among children who could not be helped by modern anticonvulsant medications,

- 27% of the 150 children had their seizures controlled or virtually controlled after 1 year on the ketogenic diet: 7% were completely free of seizures, and an additional 20% had a greater than 90% reduction.

- Half (50%) had a 50% or better decrease in their seizures.

It is notable that virtually all those remaining on the diet for 1 year had at least a 50% decrease in seizures. Those who had less than a 50% reduction often decided that the diet was too much trouble and discontinued it.

It is also noteworthy that most children who had success with the diet had shown some success during the first 3 months (see Table 3.3). The degree of success might improve after 3 months, but if a 50% decrease in seizures did not occur during that time, it was less likely to occur in subsequent months. The results appear as good as those from earlier eras, despite starting with children who have failed six—often new—medications and who were having an average of 600 seizures per month.

TABLE 3.3

Outcome of 150 Children Started on the Classic Ketogenic Diet at Hopkins in 1998

	At Onset	3 months	12 months	3–6 years later
Number	150		83	Same 83
Seizure free	0	4	11	11 off diet, 9 off meds, 8 seizure free, 2 90–99% free
90–99% free	0	46	30	23 off diet, 9 off meds, 10 seizure free, 13 90–99% free
50–90% free	0	39	34	26 off diet, 11 off meds, 2 seizure free, 6 90–99% free, 15 50–90% free
< 50% free	0	36	8	all off diet
Continued on diet		125	83	18

COMPARE THESE RESULTS with the fact that if a child's epilepsy has not been controlled with the first two medications used, that child has only a 30–40% chance of controlling his or her epilepsy with any further medication.

What is even more amazing is that 3 to 6 years after starting the diet, 13% of these 150 children were seizure free, and another 10% had only infrequent seizures. Most of these children had also been able to discontinue their anticonvulsant medications.

We even have children that have stayed on the ketogenic diet for more than 10 years. Most are seizure free or nearly so, and many are medication free. Some have tried to come off the diet and had their seizures worsen, so the diet was continued. Over time, they have found the diet relatively easy to do.

"But it has never been shown to be effective in a blinded trial" was a common complaint in the past. The difficulties of designing such a study of a diet are clear. However, two such blinded studies have been performed, and both were published since the last edition of this book. In one, by Neal, Cross, and colleagues, 103 children with at least 7 seizures per week who had failed at least 2 medications were randomly either started immediately on the diet or started after a 3-month delay. After 3 months, those in the ketogenic treatment group had a 75% decrease in their seizures compared to the control group, and 38% had a greater than 50% reduction.

In a double-blinded crossover study performed at Johns Hopkins, 20 children with the Lennox-Gastaut syndrome and a minimum of 15 drop seizures per day were randomly entered into a blinded protocol. All were begun on the classical ketogenic diet, but half, chosen randomly, were given fluids with glucose added to negate the ketosis; the remainder received saccharin-flavored fluids. After the sixth day the children were re-fasted and again begun on the diet but with the opposite fluid. Drop seizures were recorded by the parents, and these seizures were recorded also on 24-hour EEGs at the end of each phase. The outcomes are shown in Table 3.4.

Table 3.4 shows seizures (clinical events) and electroencephalography (EEG) events after interventions and at 6 and 12 months. It gives the mean number of events at baseline and after fasting and the ketogenic diet with addition of glucose or saccharin. In Figure 3.1, note the marked decrease in seizures after fasting with or without the addition of glucose and the decrease in EEG events. Note also the status at 6 and 12 months.

These two studies presented in Tables 3.3 and 3.4, although different in design, both confirm the effectiveness of the ketogenic diet in controlling difficult-to-control seizures. The old argument that there are no controlled studies about the diet is no longer true. It is rare nowadays that an insurance company will try to reject payment for the diet when these studies and the vast evidence are presented to them.

In summary, the ketogenic diet has come a long way since its discovery in the 1920s and its rediscovery in the 1990s. It is now established that carbohydrate restriction, whether with the classical ketogenic diet or one of its variations—the modified Atkins diet, the MCT diet, or the LGIT—all are effective in decreasing most types of seizures and may prove effective in the treatments of other conditions as well. If you are interested in the latest up-to-date research about ketogenic diet efficacy, go to www.epilepsy.com/ketonews, where the most recent studies are profiled, including an annual "Top 10" list of the most exciting studies.

The rest of Section I covers more specific details of why the diet works, who it works best for, and how to make it work for *you* and your family!

TABLE 3.4 Outcomes from a Randomized Trial of the Diet at Johns Hopkins (2009)

Outcome	No. patients	Spells/day prior to diet	Median decrease	Minimum/maximum	P value
Push-button events*	20	28	14.5	-14, 52	0.001
EEG events**	20	26	22.5	-112, 517	0.029

Note. *Push-button events were drop seizures recorded by parents. **EEG events were correlates of drop seizures as read by a blinded EEG reader of 24-hour EEGs.

Source: From The Ketogenic Diet: Additional Information From a Crossover Study. Freeman, JM J Child Neurol. 2009;24:509–512.

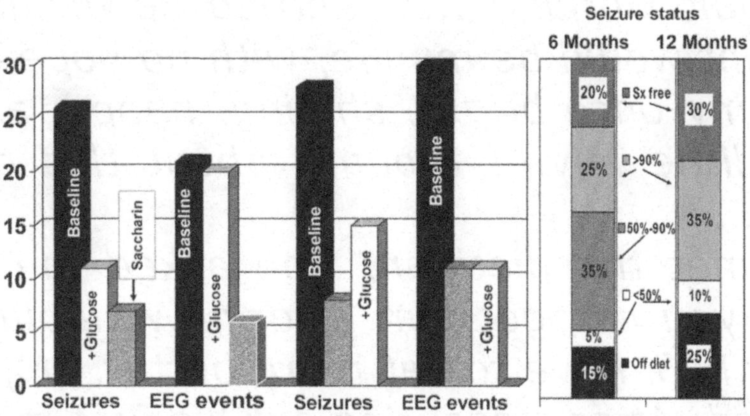

FIGURE 3.1 Seizures (clinical events) and EEG events after interventions and at 6 and 12 months. Note. Mean number of events at baseline and after fasting and the ketogenic diet with addition of glucose or saccharin. Note the marked decrease in seizures after fasting with or without addition of glucose and less decrease in EEG events. Note seizure status at 6 and 12 months.

In January, Daniel had his first tonic-clonic seizure. In the months since then, he has had thousands of seizures. Drop attacks, "jerk" episodes, staring episodes, and more tonic-clonic seizures. I stopped counting when he hit 70 in any particular day. We met our doctor, who from the beginning told me that the ketogenic diet was certainly an option, but she wanted to try medication first.

Try medication we did! Topamax®, Dilantin, Ativan, Keppra, Klonopin, and Zonegran, two of which caused nasty rashes ... I had a zom-

bie-like child on my hands who was still seizing. And things got worse. I pulled him out of day-care and quit working ... I settled down into what I thought would be my life, with no hope of getting back my once bright, shining, happy, and intelligent little boy. I thought about this diet some more...

I met the dietitian. She asked me, "Do you think you can get him to drink whipping cream? If not he'll have to eat more butter." My stomach lurched. After measuring out his first meal (which took 45 minutes), I cried like I've never cried before. But somehow we got through it, and the next morning he had only five seizures. Five!!! The next day was even better.

He has been on the diet 20 days now. He has not had a seizure in 2 weeks. I know that you've heard stories like ours before. I know that we are one of the lucky ones. I am writing to say thank you for helping me to get my son back.

CHAPTER FOUR

How Does the Ketogenic Diet Work?

This chapter was written by James Rubenstein and reviewed and updated by Dr. Adam Hartman, who is studying the ketogenic diet in animal models.

We still do not really know yet how the ketogenic diet works, despite the volume of work that has been done since the last edition of our book was published 4 years ago. Being able to answer this crucial question involves a better understanding of three *factors* that occur when an individual has a seizure: onset of the event; the spreading of the seizure through the brain, which determines the type of seizure that will occur; and how cessation of the seizure occurs. Starting a patient on the ketogenic diet essentially tricks the body into thinking it is maintaining a fasting state. The body is denied most carbohydrates, is given sufficient protein, and depending upon the dietary ratio chosen by the dietitian for the individual patient, is given large amounts of fat. The body quickly depletes it's supply of easily accessed carbohydrate as it turns to fat as its alternative energy source. Fasting accelerates the process, and as fats are burned without the presence of carbohydrates, ketone bodies accumulate and can be identified and measured in the blood, urine, and cerebral spinal fluid. The simplest way to identify if an individual has a large ketone supply on board is simply to smell the fruity aroma on the individual's breath. It is very dramatic.

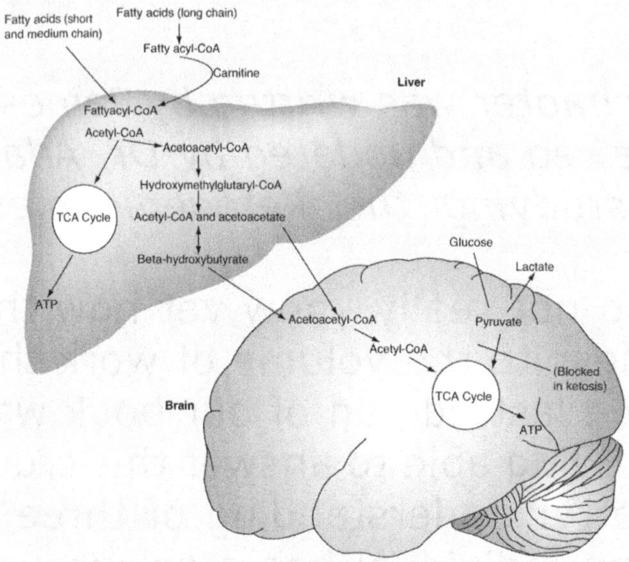

FIGURE 4.1 Breakdown of fatty acids into ketones by the liver and update by the brain for energy.

KETONES

Once the ketogenic diet is established, there are ketone bodies available to cross the blood–brain barrier and enter the brain. Once they are in there, we don't know exactly what happens, but it's clear that there can be a significant effect on one of the three factors mentioned previously (onset, propagation, and/or cessation of the seizures).

There are three types of ketone bodies, which are water-soluble compounds produced as the byproducts of burning fat for energy instead of carbohydrate. They are called acetone, acetoacetate, and betahydroxybutyrate. We still do not know if any of them, or which ones, are somehow responsible for improving seizure control. They may just be *indicators* of the presence of some other factors or metabolic changes that we have not yet identified that are the key.

It also has been proposed that somehow the entire mystery is related to the way the body produces or uses insulin as it moves from burning primarily carbohydrate to burning primarily fat.

Because the ketone bodies are acids and cause acidosis (an increase in the amount of acid in the body), it has been proposed that the ketogenic diet works by creating an ongoing acidotic state that the body somehow compensates for, while it is also affecting one of the three factors. This was one of the first theories, but it has been largely disproven.

We know that once the body realizes that a certain level of ketones are circulating in the blood, they "spill" into the urine and can be measured there. However, that does not always seem to correlate with the actual amount of ketone bodies in the bloodstream. Levels of the ketone bodies in the blood and urine do not have a strong correlation with their levels in the brains of rodents (the brian, of course, is where the seizures are taking place) but as of now, we do not have a way to reliably measure these changes in people. Studies that have attempted to link blood (or urine) ketones with seizure control have not shown a consistent link. Many researchers believe that ketosis is a marker that indicates that your body has made the metabolic shift to be on the ketogenic diet, but they do not necessarily believe that ketosis is exactly *why* the diet works.

ANIMAL MODELS

Researchers have continued to expand their work with different types of animal models. They can now evaluate the efficacy of a drug (medication) or a metabolic treatment (such as the ketogenic diet, the Modified Atkins Diet, or the Low Glycemic Index Treatment) in altering the frequency of seizures.

One of the challenges in studying how the ketogenic diet works in animals is that, surprisingly, the diet does not work well in most standard animal seizure tests. It does work in two of them in mice (the 6Hz test, which models partial-onset seizures, and the fluorothyl test, which models generalized seizures) and one in rats (pentylenetetrazol, which identifies medicines that work in absence and myoclonic seizures). It also works in some chemical and electrical kindling models, which induce both generalized and partial seizure types.

We know that there are a number of channels (proteins that allow transport of molecules across the cell membrane) in the brain that are affected by seizures, as well as the drugs and diets used to treat them. Examples you are probably familiar with include the Ca++(calcium), K+(potassium), and GABA (gaba-amino-butyric acid) channels. Somehow, these channels and others may be the actual *regulators* of brain electrical activity, and understanding how they affect the three factors may ultimately determine how the ketogenic diet and other dietary therapies work.

Other, newer animal models to study the three factors, and hence how the ketogenic diet works, are being created by hyperthermia (drastically altering temperature), brain trauma, hypoxia (lack of oxygen), vascular occlusion (similar to a stroke), radiation exposure, chemical exposure causing brain toxicity, and genetic alterations where genes are removed or replaced, called *genetically modified, transgenic, knock-out,* or *knock-in* mice.

The animal can be studied clinically, but there are also methods for studying how brain slices and cultures of brain tissue in the variously altered models react to different treatment modalities. By pursuing a large variety of possible models, it can be expected that one or more of them will yield different details to explain the three factors and then to also explain the way both dietary and pharmacologic treatments work.

THE FUTURE

In the near future, you are likely to read more about

- the effect of chronic ketosis on brain energy reserves and mitochondria, the cell's powerhouse;
- how ketosis alters the utilization of glutamic acid (an excitatory amino acid that promotes seizures) and GABA (an inhibitory amino acid that stops seizures);
- how the ketogenic diet alters various neurotransmitter levels, which may play a role in explaining the efficacy of the ketogenic diet not only in treating seizures but also in treating a variety of other neurological and behavioral disorders;
- the role of the diet in the levels of PUFAs (polyunsaturated fatty acids), which are known to modulate neuronal hyperexcitability;
- the role of adenosine and other neuromodulators in the mechanisms of action of the diet;
- whether fasting is the same as (or likely different than) the diet;
- the relative role of glucose stabilization versus high fats (with studies examining a drug currently called 2-DG that helps stabilize glucose and may help reduce seizures); and
- the importance of cellular metabolism-sensing pathways (in either neurons or their supporting cells) in altering sensitivity to seizures.

Unfortunately, our inability to explain exactly how the diet works has led many pediatric neurologists to remain skeptical, and some still remain quite negative about its potential usefulness. There have been studies that suggest that the ketogenic diet ranks about 14th on many physicians' lists of effective seizure treatments, despite the known fact that if a child has failed two medications used appropriately, the ketogenic diet has a greater likelihood of achieving more than 50% seizure reduction than the next medication introduced. We tell these child neurologists that we do not know how many medications work either, initially, including Keppra® (levetiracetam), which is now one of the most popular drugs! The diet, just like many medications, probably has multiple mechanisms of action. Finally, basic scientists are working together with clinical researchers to find ways to make the diet more effective in humans.

CHAPTER FIVE

Is My Child a Candidate for the Ketogenic Diet?

Perhaps the most common question asked of us by parents is whether or not we believe the ketogenic diet is likely to be helpful for their child. Quoting the odds is great, but because every child is different, is there a way to know who will respond and who will not? Most of the anticonvulsant medicines on the market now are initially used for partial (focal) seizures, and of course always in adults first. As most parents are no doubt aware, as time and familiarity with new drugs occurs, these medicines are used not only for generalized seizures (which involve the entire brain all at once) but in young children as well. Sometimes figuring this out takes years. What about the ketogenic diet, which has been used for nearly a century now? For whom does it work best? When should it be tried? Who is it unlikely to help? The answers to these questions are becoming clearer as the diet is being used more.

WHEN IN THE COURSE OF EPILEPSY?

In general, the diet is used for children with intractable seizures, often occurring daily, that have failed at least two medications for seizure control.

Does this mean the diet wouldn't be helpful earlier? Definitely not, and we suspect the opposite. For more information about using the diet first-line, read Chapter 24.

When compared to many anticonvulsants, especially those of the *older* generation (e.g., phenobarbital, Dilantin®, Depakote®, Tegretol®), the diet, in our opinion, has a better side-effect profile. When compared to many of the newer drugs, the diet is certainly better established with more data, especially in kids, to support its use. In our experience as well, we do not see the same potential side effects. So why isn't the diet used first? There is no doubt that it is easier to take a pill than to restrict calories, carbohydrates, and fluids and change the entire family's lifestyle with the ketogenic diet. However, there is nothing worse than seeing a child for a second opinion that has failed over 10 medications over many years who was not offered the ketogenic diet as an option. The diet should be offered earlier in the course of epilepsy in children, and many epilepsy centers agree. The same feeling is the subject of research into an earlier use of other therapies such as surgery and the vagus nerve stimulator.

Sandra was a 5-year-old girl with new onset of frequent complex partial seizures. Her brother Charlie was on the ketogenic diet for 4 years, having come to see us after years of difficult-to-control seizures that didn't respond to any medications. Charlie had a dramatic response to the diet and was taken off the diet mostly due to a lack of seizures than any other reason. Due to Charlie's success, the family wanted to try the diet before any other medications were tried. Although this was an unusual request, Sandra was started on the diet and did just as well as her brother. Because Sandra's parents had lots of experience with the diet, it made the change in lifestyle much easier for Sandra to handle.

WHO IS LIKELY TO BE A SUPER-RESPONDER TO THE DIET?

In general, we don't know for sure. Parents often come to Johns Hopkins to be started on the diet after they see a video, television special, or newspaper article that highlights an amazing "miracle" responder to the ketogenic diet. These children start the diet, are seizure-free within 1–2 weeks (sometimes after the fast), and are medication-free within months. Although wonderful to take care of, these children are uncommon (probably about 10% of our patients on the diet). Based on our information from 1998, more than one-quarter of patients will have a 90% or greater reduction in seizures, but all seizure types appeared to be equally likely to respond. Younger age tended to do slightly better as well.

A few years ago, we looked at 3 years of ketogenic diet patients to see who the "super-responders" were. We found out the same thing as we did years ago:

All seizure types, ages, weights, and severities of seizures of children were likely to be miracle responders. The only exceptions were children with *just* complex partial (focal) seizures, many of whom were possible surgery candidates but chose to try the diet first. This is not to say that many children with partial seizures don't do well on the diet; many had 90% or greater seizure reductions and were able to lower medicines, but the diet is rarely a cure in this situation. In this situation, if the diet is tried and ineffective after 3 to 6 months, and surgery is an option, we would suggest surgery be looked into at an epilepsy center.

In this study, there were only a few children with Doose syndrome (myoclonic-astatic epilepsy). Our suspicion was that if we did this study again, now years later, this syndrome would turn out to be one in which children are likely to be super-responders. In fact, we often tell families of children in which this is a possible diagnosis that the response to the ketogenic diet is the best "test" for Doose syndrome we know. Keep reading for more information about Doose syndrome.

SPECIAL DISORDERS

All that aside, we have our beliefs, based on very recent information, that certain neurologic conditions do extremely well on the diet. Some of this research is from our center, some from others, and some combined. This list is by no means complete but does influence when we decide to try the diet earlier with some patients. These conditions are the perhaps most important. (For more information, see Table 1 of the 2009 international ketogenic diet consensus paper.)

Infantile spasms

In 2002, we published our experience using the diet for infants with one of the most terrifying epilepsy disorders: infantile spasms (West syndrome). In this condition, infants around 6 months of age develop the sudden onset of clustering body jerks, often out of sleep, with a chaotic EEG, and occasional loss of developmental skills. Treatments include ACTH and vigabatrin, but these drugs have serious side effects, and vigabatrin requires lots of paperwork in order to prescribe nowadays. Knowing the diet can be provided via an infant formula and has fewer side effects, it's a natural choice. We found that nearly half of the 23 children we had treated, usually those with tough-to-control infantile spasms, had a 90% or better response, improvement on EEG, and better development by 6 months. Infants under age 1 year and who had failed no more than three drugs did better.

Based on this, we have now more than doubled our use of the ketogenic diet for infantile spasms and are seeing the same results—we have treated 2010, by 104 children with infantile spasms. About two-thirds will have a >90% reduction in spasms.

We are also using the diet for new-onset infantile spasms (rather than steroids or vigabatrin).

Alexander was a 6-month-old baby when he developed infantile spasms. After initially responding to ACTH, his seizures returned and didn't go away with a second round of ACTH. Alexander then tried three other medications before starting the ketogenic diet. Although his spasms did not vanish on the diet, they were reduced from 10 clusters a day to 2, and his EEG improved. Best of all, his alertness and development improved as well. He remained on the diet for 2 years total and is now only on a single drug.

MYOCLONIC-ASTATIC (DOOSE) EPILEPSY

In this disorder, children (often ages 3–5 years) present with the sudden onset of head drop seizures and occasionally cognitive decline. Although many neurologists think this is Lennox-Gastaut syndrome, the EEG often shows periods of normal background making this less likely. Traditional medicines such as Depakote® and Keppra® are only occasionally useful. We have used the ketogenic diet for about a dozen of these children with occasionally dramatic success. Allie is one such child, and her story is even highlighted on our epilepsy center's Web site as a sidebar. Allie became seizure-free within 2 weeks of starting the diet, and her medications were stopped quickly after. Several patients with likely Doose epilepsy have also been similar responders on the modified Atkins diet. Dr. Douglas Nordli from Chicago and Dr. Sudha Kessler from Philadelphia have also seen this improvement with patients having Doose epilepsy, and both have published their experience in medical journals. For more information, go to http://www.doosesyndrome.com.

TUBEROUS SCLEROSIS COMPLEX

In a combined study from Johns Hopkins and the Massachusetts General Hospital, we found 12 children with tuberous sclerosis complex (multiple brain tubers; ash-leaf spots on the skin; heart and kidney tubers; epilepsy) that were started on the ketogenic diet did very well. Many had a history of infantile spasms in the past, but none at the time of starting the diet. All but one child had half their seizures improve, and half had >90% improvement. Five children even had several months seizure free. Although there are a limited number of patients, Dr. Elizabeth Thiele and our group agree that the ketogenic diet is a good option for patients with tuberous sclerosis complex. Interestingly, at least in our experience, having this condition also made it more likely for seizures to come back in those children who became seizure free on the diet (sometimes years later). In that way, it's possible that although the diet is a big help for tuberous sclerosis, it may be a more long-term treatment than for Doose syndrome or certainly infantile spasms.

GLUT-1 TRANSPORTER DEFICIENCY

In this rare condition, the molecule that allows glucose to cross into the brain to be used as fuel is missing. Children will often have seizures and cognitive delay until this is recognized, most often by noticing a very low glucose level in the spinal fluid after a spinal tap. Logically, if the body cannot use glucose, then fat makes sense as a better alternative fuel. The ketogenic diet is considered the first and only therapy of choice for children with GLUT-1. More information for this disorder can be found on the internet and in Chapter 24.

GASTROSTOMY TUBE OR INFANT-FORMULA–FED CHILDREN

Perhaps one of the easiest groups of children to place on the ketogenic diet are those who do not eat solid foods. If the diet is given just as liquids, it avoids all compliance issues. Infants on formula or are breastfeeding will need to directly switch to one of several ketogenic formulas (see Chapter 8 for instructions), which can then be continued for months to years. As infants turn into toddlers, small amounts of solid ketogenic baby foods can be introduced after 1–2 months. Children that are fed using gastrostomy tubes (G-tubes) can also be started on the diet without compliance issues. In a study performed at Johns Hopkins, since 1998, more than a quarter of all patients started on the diet did so using formula only. Nearly 60% had a >90% improvement in seizures, double the average ketogenic diet patient. In any child in an intensive care setting for epilepsy, the diet can be easily started or continued via a temporary nasogastric tube.

The formulas available are very palatable with a taste similar to most other infant formulas. It is easy to calculate for the dietitian and can be soy-based, milk-based, or even hypoallergenic. There is also less room for error and less education involved for parents. The presence of a gastrostomy tube also allows medications to be provided without carbohydrate sweeteners or flavoring. Patients who are ill on the ketogenic diet can occasionally have acidosis and dehydration, but having a gastrostomy tube helps avoid this. Lastly, insurance companies often cover formula in children with gastrostomy tubes because it is being used as a medical therapy rather than for solely nutritional purposes.

Kaylee was a 9-year-old girl with cerebral palsy and daily drop seizures. For years she had a gastrostomy tube for her nutrition and was fed continuously at night only. After failing to achieve seizure control with Keppra and Lamictal, her parents asked to try the ketogenic diet. During the ketogenic diet admission week, switching from Pediasure to KetoCal ® was easy for her parents to do and did not cost them any more money per month. Within 2 weeks her seizures were significantly reduced, and the family did not find the diet much different than her previous formula, except for the occasional lab work and checking urine ketones.

OTHER CONDITIONS

There are several other conditions in which the diet may be very helpful. They include Dravet syndrome, absence epilepsy, Rett syndrome, Lennox-Gastaut syndrome, and mitochondrial disorders. In these conditions, several articles have reported the ketogenic diet as leading to superb results. There are conditions, however, in which the diet is not a good idea. These conditions are presented in the following list, which is reproduced in part from the 2009 consensus statement.

Contraindications to the use of the ketogenic diet:

Absolute

Carnitine deficiency (primary)

Carnitine palmitoyltransferase (CPT) I or II deficiency

Carnitine translocase deficiency

ß-oxidation defects

Medium-chain acyl dehydrogenase deficiency (MCAD)

Long-chain acyl dehydrogenase deficiency (LCAD)

Short-chain acyl dehydrogenase deficiency (SCAD)

Long-chain 3-hydroxyacyl-CoA deficiency

Medium-chain 3-hydroxyacyl-CoA deficiency

Pyruvate car+boxylase deficiency

Porphyria

Relative

Inability to maintain adequate nutrition

Surgical focus identified by neuroimaging and video-EEG monitoring

Parent or caregiver noncompliance

DOES AGE MATTER?

Probably not, but there is a slight trend toward improved seizure control in younger children (see Table 5.1). Younger children often can maintain high ketosis for long periods and compliance is less of a problem. We feel, as do other doctors, that infants may be one of the ideal groups for the diet for this reason. They certainly need extra care due to growth issues, but can do very well on the diet.

What about adolescents and adults? Most centers will tell parents that the diet is impossible to do for a teenager. In a study from both our group and Dr. James Wheless's at the University of Texas at Houston, we combined our teenage population on the diet (45 teens in total) and found that compliance was very good, seizure reduction was similar to younger children, and side effects were low. Of the participants, 44% were able to stick it out for a year. Menstrual irregularities happened in almost half of teenage girls, but this is tough to separate out from the normal irregularities of this age and the effects of medications. In general, at present we tend to use the modified Atkins diet for most teenagers.

TABLE 5.1 The Effect of Age on Outcomes of the Ketogenic Diet

Age at Start of Diet	# Initiating Diet	>50% Control at 12 Months
< 2 years	N=27	59% (1 seizure free)
2–5 years	N=50	56% (4 seizure free)
5–8 years	N=32	50% (4 seizure free)
8–12 years	N=25	40% (1 seizure free)
> 12 years	N=16	31% (1 seizure free)
Total	N=150	50% (11 seizure free)

Source: Adapted from Freeman et al., Pediatrics, 1998.

Dr. Michael Sperling, Dr. Maromei Nei, and their group of epilepsy specialists at the Jefferson Medical College in Philadelphia have used the diet for adults for years, with good results. Cholesterol does increase, and compliance can be an issue, but ketosis occurs and seizures often improve. We also mostly use the modified Atkins diet here at Johns Hopkins for adults over age 18 years, and we have had good results.

> *Jack was a 34-year-old man from Ohio with intractable seizures. After failing to see any improvement with a temporal lobe resection, he became interested in alternative approaches. Herbs and biofeedback failed to help his seizures, so he found our center over the internet and enrolled in our Atkins diet study for adults. After 3 months, his seizures had dropped from five per month to two, and he was making moderate ketones consistently. However, he was unprepared for how difficult the diet would be to follow and decided to stop. Interestingly, since that time his seizures have remained somewhat improved.*

INTELLIGENCE

The level of a child's intelligence is not a criterion for selecting appropriate candidates for the diet. Some of the most dramatic successes have occurred in the most profoundly handicapped children. Other successes have occurred in children with normal intelligence. However, it is important for parents to carefully assess their goals and expectations before starting the diet. Parents may believe that their child's substantial intellectual delay is due solely to the medications and that if they could only get their child off medication everything would be back to normal. Such parents are likely to be disappointed.

On the other hand, *electrical* seizures may be even more frequent than *clinical* seizures and may indeed interfere with intellect. Children with frequent myoclonic or *drop* seizures may have very chaotic EEGs and may have had intellectual deterioration since the start of their seizures. Such children may experience striking intellectual improvement if the diet is effective in controlling their seizures.

In short, the diet is intended primarily to control seizures. Decreasing and discontinuing medications is certainly important, but only a secondary goal. Improving intellect is a hope and a desire, but that is not what the ketogenic diet is designed to do.

TIME COMMITMENT

One of the only things that truly will lead to diet failure is a lack of commitment and time to make it work, which can be both the fault of the family and the physicians. The diet requires a significant investment of the *entire* family to spend a week to start and learn the diet in the hospital, calculate meal plans and weigh foods, and avoid cheating. A family in which the parents are divorced and one parent does not believe in the diet will nearly always be a ketogenic diet failure. Similarly, if grandparents or other caregivers do not agree that the diet is worth trying and make meals for children that will sabotage the diet, obviously this will not work.

Giving the diet at least 1–2 months to work before making any big medication changes is also crucial.

Close communication with the physician and dietitian is not only a good idea, it's mandatory to make the diet work. The hospital team also must spend considerable time and energy to make the diet program effective with email and phone contact with families, handling illnesses and providing support, and watching and monitoring for both expected and unexpected problems.

CHAPTER SIX

The Diet for All Cultures, Religions, Food Preferences, and Allergies

MY CHILD IS ON A GLUTEN-FREE DIET. CAN THE KETOGENIC DIET BE DONE? WHAT ABOUT IF WE ARE VEGETARIAN?

The ketogenic diet can be used for all different cultures and food restrictions. It is used in all continents except Antarctica. In China, Japan, and Korea, it is growing incredibly in popularity. Similarly, in India, it is also becoming widely used.

Many parents would think that it would be impossible to try a diet that already limits many of their child's favorite foods; however the ketogenic diet can be used for any child that has gastrointestinal restrictions, allergies, preferences, or follows any diet for religious reasons. Prior to diet initiation, it is important for the parents to inform the doctor or dietitian seeing the patient of all the child's allergies or religious food restrictions.

KOSHER

Keeping kosher is a set of biblical dietary restrictions that many observant Jewish people follow. The word *kosher* is Hebrew and means fit, proper, or correct. The diet consists of restricting certain foods like pork and shellfish, and not mixing certain foods together like milk and meat. Due to these restrictions many foods have certifications from Rabbis to identify that the food is kosher.

When people see pictures of the ketogenic diet, they think of a lot of butter, cream, and hot dogs. When eating kosher, because hot dogs are meat they cannot be eaten with butter or cream, which are both dairy. However, there are many substitutions for either the dairy products or the meat products.

> *Noah is a 5-year-old male with Doose syndrome. Prior to starting the diet he was on a regular kosher diet. He ate three meals and two snacks averaging 1,200 calories per day. He has always had normal growth. His parents were very concerned about starting the ketogenic diet while maintaining their religious beliefs and keeping a kosher diet. A closer look at Noah's diet showed he liked all proteins, including eggs, cheese, chicken, ground beef, and turkey; he liked a lot of carbohydrates, but he was not much of a milk*

drinker. By reviewing with the parents what foods cannot be mixed together and finding foods that are pareve, *those that can be combined with the meat or dairy meals, the dietitian was able to come with a meal plan.*

Noah did very well on the ketogenic diet and was seizure-free within the first 2 weeks of starting the diet. With the help of ketogenic diet computer programs, Noah's parents were able to use their kosher brands of foods and make it work on the ketogenic diet.

SAMPLE KOSHER MEAL PLAN

Breakfast	Lunch	Dinner
eggs	kosher turkey deli	kosher roasted chicken coated with macadamia nuts
kosher American cheese	mayo	egg
butter	olive oil (mixed with mayo)	oil
cream	tomato	spinach
applesauce	lettuce	margarine
	avocado	

Snacks

peanut butter and margarine

"keto yogurt" (sour cream, heavy cream, and fruit)

Currently the only kosher formula on the market is the modular version with RCF®, Microlipid®, and Polycose®. KetoVolve®, although not on the U.S. market at time of publication, claims it will be kosher certified.

HALAL

Halal is an Arabic word meaning permitted or lawful. Halal is a term that applies to all facets of Muslim life, including food. All foods are considered Halal except for pork, alcohol, carnivorous animals, animals that were improperly slaughtered, and any food product containing any of the mentioned products. Starting the ketogenic diet while keeping the laws of Halal is not difficult; all you need to do is obtain the food values for each product, and each product can be added to the computer program to calculate the meals. A meal plan for a child who only eats Halal would be very similar to the kosher meal, however, someone who eats only Halal can mix milk and meat together and have cream or butter mixed into their foods.

ALLERGIES

There are many children with food allergies or intolerances. Your child could be allergic to only milk or have multiple food allergies consisting of milk, soy, eggs, wheat, and nuts. You might wonder how your child could go on a restrictive diet when you already have to restrict his or her diet.

Jake was allergic to milk, soy, eggs, nuts, and chicken when his mother was considering the ketogenic diet. After being informed about the diet, she looked up online what the diet entails and saw on every site recipes that consist of eggs, cream, and butter. Jake's mother called the doctor to say that she was unsure if Jake could go on the diet with his multiple food allergies. When we spoke to Jake's mom, she sat down with us and reviewed Jake's current intake. He was eating baby food beef mixed with baby food vegetables or fruit, coconut milk, and coconut butter. We informed Jake's mother that going on the diet was not going to change his diet that much. He could still eat his baby food meats, fruit, and vegetables, and now they would be mixed with coconut oils or milk.

The trick with allergies is to look at what the child is currently eating, and pair it with a fat that they can tolerate. There are so many options out there now for patients that have allergies that it is not difficult at all.

Milk Allergies

Ingredients to avoid:

butter, butter fat, butter milk
casein
cheese
cottage cheese

curds
cream
custard
pudding
ghee
half and half
lactalbumin
lactalbumin phosphate
lactoglobulin
lactose
nougat
rennet casein
sour cream
sour cream solids
yogurt

For high fat keto replacements:

1. instead of butter, try margarine;
2. instead of cream, try coconut milk; and
3. remember, mayonnaise and oils are both dairy free.

Egg Allergies

Read the labels and avoid:

albumin
egg yolk
egg powder
egg substitutes
globulin

egg white
dried egg
egg solids
eggnog
livetin
mayonnaise
meringue
ovomucin
ovovitellin
lysozyme (used in Europe)
ovalbumin
ovomucoid
simplesse

To replace an egg needed for baking, one of the following may be substituted in recipes; however, each ingredient needs to be calculated for each recipe, and they still do not provide enough protein.

- 1tsp baking powder, 1tbsp water, 1tbsp vinegar
- 1tsp yeast dissolved in 1/4 cup warm water
- 1tbsp apricot puree
- 1 1/2tbsp water, 1 1/2tbsp oil, 1tsp baking powder
- 1 packet gelatin, 2tbsp warm water (do not mix until ready to use)

Soy Allergy

Ingredients to avoid:

hydrolyzed soy protein
miso
shoyo sauce

soy flour
soy grits
soy nuts
soy milk
soy sprouts
soy protein concentrate
soy protein isolate
soy sauce
tempeh
textured vegetable protein (TVP)
tofu

And watch these products because they may contain soy:

flavorings
hydrolyzed plant protein
hydrolyzed vegetable protein
natural flavoring
vegetable broth
vegetable gum
vegetable starch

Peanuts and Tree Nut Allergies

Peanuts and tree nuts are high in fat and a good source of protein, which is why they are found in a lot of ketogenic recipes; however, they are not an essential part of the ketogenic diet and can be eliminated.

Ingredients to avoid:

almonds
arachis oil
Brazil nuts
cashews
chestnuts
hazelnuts (filberts)
gianduja
hickory nuts
Macadamia nuts
marzipan/almond paste
nougat
Nu-Nuts®
artificial nuts
nut butters
nut oil
nut paste
pecans
pine nuts (pignolia, pinian)
pistachios
peanuts
peanut butter
peanut flour
walnuts
cold pressed, expressed, or expelled peanut oil

Wheat Allergies

A wheat allergy is actually very easy on the ketogenic diet because most products containing wheat are very high in carbohydrates. However, there are some food products that have wheat in them that you would not expect.

Ingredients to avoid

food thickeners
gelatinized starch
hydrolyzed vegetable protein
meat and crab substitutes
modified food starch
natural flavoring
soy sauce
starch
vegetable gum
vegetable starch

Children with any allergy or multiple allergies should have no issue going on the ketogenic diet. However, there must be a long conversation among the doctor, dietitian, and family about the allergies and food intolerances.

Sample Meal Plan for Multiple Food Allergies

Breakfast: coconut pancake (coconut flour, coconut oil, flaxseed, coconut milk, baking powder, gelatin)

Lunch: chicken, avocado, canola oil, coconut milk, and spinach

Dinner: salmon, butternut squash, canola oil, and coconut milk

Snack: bacon, canola oil, McDonalds french fries, coconut milk, and fruit

For children that have multiple food allergies and require a formula, a modular formula needs to be used. If the child is allergic to only milk, then RCF®, Polycose®, and Microlipid® can be used. If the child has multiple food allergies, then Complete Amino Acid® mix is used instead of RCF®. Complete Amino Acid® mix is just the essential proteins and does not contain any vitamins and minerals.

GLUTEN-FREE, CASEIN-FREE

There are many children who follow a gluten-free, casein-free diet for autism or behavioral issues. Gluten is a protein found in wheat, rye, and barley and is the material in flours that acts like a glue and holds the dough together. Maintaining a gluten-free diet on the ketogenic diet is not difficult because gluten is found in foods that are high in carbohydrates. Casein is also a protein found in milk products. Therefore, all cheeses, yogurts, and any product containing milk are avoided.

Children on a gluten-free, casein-free diet before starting the ketogenic diet will follow a diet similar for those with a milk allergy. All dairy is removed and replaced with nondairy items, such as margarine and oils.

VEGETARIAN

There are many different types of vegetarianism, and people choose to follow a vegetarian lifestyle for multiple reasons. The most restricted form of vegetarianism is a vegan diet, which omits all animal products from a diet. While following a vegan diet, the most concerning nutritional issue is protein intake; nevertheless, there are multiple ways to take in adequate protein by eating beans or eating meat or fish substitutes while on a regular vegan diet.

The issue with following a vegan diet while on the ketogenic diet is that beans and meat substitutes are usually high in carbohydrates as opposed to an animal protein like chicken, which has zero carbohydrates. However, there are protein powders available that could be added to meal plans of cream, fruit or vegetable, and oils and margarine.

If a family chooses to follow any other form of vegetarianism, such as lacto ovo or pescetarian, usually omit only 1–2 types of animal protein and eat all of the others.

ORGANIC

Many families choose to buy only organic foods, both produce and prepared foods. This is a choice made by the family. There are no studies indicating increased seizure reduction while eating an organic diet, however, many people believe that the food is better for you. There are no contraindications to following a completely organic diet while on the ketogenic diet.

SUMMARY

It is important for parents and clinicians to realize that the ketogenic diet can be done with all different types of diets. The most important thing is to look at what the child is eating prior to starting the diet, and figure out a way that fats can be added to what that child currently eats. If the child has an allergy, then look at the foods that he is currently eating and figure out how to add in the fat. Are the parents going to mix oil with mayonnaise? Can they mix coconut oil into the baby foods? If these or similar questions can be answered positively, then that child can start the ketogenic diet and will be very successful. It's up to the parents to be enthusiastic about the foods, and it's up to the clinicians to encourage and support the parents and patient while they are evaluating which foods will fit into their lifestyle.

SECTION II

The ABCs of the Ketogenic Diet

CHAPTER SEVEN

Initiating the Ketogenic Diet: To Fast or Admit?

At Johns Hopkins, initiating the ketogenic diet is a process, not an event. The journey begins before a child is accepted into the ketogenic diet program. For patients who have been seen in our pediatric epilepsy clinic, parents are informed about the diet, and its advantages and difficulties for their child are discussed. It is suggested that they read this book and become familiar with the diet before deciding to make the commitment.

Patients who live a distance from us are asked to send the child's EEG reports and other medical records for review by the staff. Parents are also asked to write a statement of expectations describing their child and their (the parents') personal goals for the diet. This statement enables us to better comprehend the parents' goals and expectations. Parents who expect a *cure* may be disappointed in some situations. Parents who desire a decrease in their child's seizure frequency or in the medication toxicity are more likely to have their goals achieved.

We have had no firm criteria for accepting or rejecting children for diet initiation at Johns Hopkins. In general, however,

- most children have more than weekly seizures;
- most children have tried at least two anticonvulsants without achieving seizure control (occasionally we will accept children whose seizures have been controlled but only at the expense of medication toxicity); and
- most parents have realistic goals and positive attitudes.

Because children with infantile spasms or Doose syndrome (a syndrome with drop seizures) as well as those with the Lennox-Gastaut pattern may be more likely to respond to the diet than to medication, we are more likely to accept them for the diet earlier in the course of their epilepsy.

> THE KETOGENIC DIET should *not* be saved for a last resort only when a child has failed multiple medications. The diet should be considered early in the course of epilepsy and possibly should be tried after two medications have failed to control the seizures.

After being scheduled for diet initiation, parents are asked to keep a seizure calendar for the month before hospitalization and to read this book. We suggest they tell their local child neurologist and pediatrician what is going to happen, especially if they live far away, because they are extended members of our team. Babysitters, caregivers, and even school nurses need to be on board for the journey.

THE ADMISSIONS PROCESS

Just before admission at Johns Hopkins (other centers may have slightly different practices), a child is evaluated as an outpatient, and the parents attend their first lesson on the history of the diet, which includes an overview of the expected course of the hospitalization.

Starting the diet at Johns Hopkins then requires 4 days of hospitalization at our center beginning with fasting and followed by the gradual introduction of the high-fat meals. (More on fasting later.) During the initial phase of the diet, which lasts several weeks, the body gradually becomes adjusted to the smaller portions and lower calorie levels of the diet, as well as to digesting the larger quantities of fat. Several weeks may be required for the child's energy level to return to normal. During this period, the family also becomes accustomed to weighing and measuring all meals and to reading food labels, and the child gradually becomes adjusted to the foods of the diet and to not eating other foods.

THE FASTING DEBATE

Does the ketogenic diet need to be done in a hospital? Is fasting required to initiate the diet? There is debate both about whether or not the ketogenic diet must be initiated in the hospital and about whether or not it needs to be begun with fasting. The ketogenic diet was originally begun by fasting patients for as long as 25 days giving only water. In the 1960s, doctors at Johns Hopkins fasted patients until they had lost 10% of their body weight, usually for 10 days. To make the diet more humane, we later developed a protocol using 48 hours of fasting, and then moved to our current protocol of just 24 hours of fasting.

We believe that the initial fast is useful. The fasting jump-starts the ketosis, and evidence would suggest the diet will work quicker (about 9 days on average) if a child is fasted. After 24 hours of fasting a child is usually in deep ketosis, and any food looks good. Gradual introduction of the diet, increasing from one-third of the prescribed amount to two-thirds and then to the full diet, enables the child to adjust to the fatty food and to achieve good ketosis (and often a reduction in seizures) before he goes home.

Is a fast absolutely necessary? Definitely not. We review all children's cases before they are admitted and decide in advance if a fast is not safe. This may be if a child is felt to be too unstable or has significant issues with dehydration or nutrition to start. Good evidence from Dr. Bergqvist and her team at Children's Hospital of Philadelphia has shown that the results are the same after 3 months, fasting or not. For most families, however, the quicker onset of seizure control is reassuring and a "bonus." We look at the 1-day fast as "IV loading" of the diet. Remember, too, that fasting doesn't limit carbohydrate-free liquids, such as diet ginger ale, Fruit2O, and water.

We introduce the diet with a "keto shake," a milkshake-like meal that is easy to calculate and that may also be frozen into keto ice cream or microwaved into creamy scrambled eggs. KetoCal® can be used for this as well. We have found that offering one-third of a regular diet meal at initiation is unattractive: It comes to a sprig of broccoli on one edge of a large plate, a thumbnail-size piece of turkey on another, and a swallow of cream. The parent's usual reaction is "Arrrgh!!" Initiating the diet with a keto shake avoids this unpleasant experience and also eliminates mistakes by our hospital's dietary service. However, there are some children who just do not like the "eggnog," no matter how hard we try! For those children, we may advance the diet to solid foods a bit earlier than the night before discharge (our usual time).

PROBLEMS WITH DIET INITIATION

When the previously described protocol is followed, we have occasionally seen children become too ketotic and begin vomiting. Reversal of this condition requires some orange juice (about 30cc or 1 ounce) to restore balance. We have rarely seen children develop symptomatic hypoglycemia, with a decreased responsiveness, sometimes pallor and sweating. This is also responsive to a small amount of orange juice. These unusual but potentially serious side effects are part of why we prefer to have children in the hospital during the diet initiation, where they can be closely observed and treated, if necessary.

Sometimes the problems at initiation are psychological. We are leery of making a mother deny food to her child for this prolonged period of time without the support of the medical staff and of other mothers. Not feeding your child is very unnatural and difficult to do.

We also find that the 4-day hospital stay gives parents the opportunity to focus on the diet, to learn how to calculate meals, and to learn the purpose of what they will be doing. We feel that the intense (at least 2 hours per day) instructional process is a key element in our success.

Have we tested each of these elements? No. Are they all necessary? We don't know. Can the diet be initiated without hospitalization? This has been done, too. If a family is able to come back for frequent classes, and they are more comfortable at home, on rare occasions we have started the diet as an outpatient without a fast, with good success. However, for the vast majority of children, at Johns Hopkins we continue with the protocol that has brought our patients such success: 4 days of hospitalization with hours of teaching each day.

On the 4th day after hospital admission, the child is discharged home. The families are ready for the journey ahead. This marks the end of the initiation process and the beginning of the *fine-tuning* phase.

FINE-TUNING THE DIET

Fine-tuning the ketogenic diet begins after discharge and is usually done by phone or email. It involves the dietitians adjusting the various components of the diet—calories, liquids, fats, recipes, ketogenic ratios, and so forth—to achieve the best level of ketosis for optimal seizure control. Fine-tuning can be an important part to achieving success on the diet for some children and is discussed further in Chapter 12.

GETTING READY FOR THE DIET: THE PARENTS' PERSPECTIVE

Psychological preparation

The most important factor contributing to the success of the ketogenic diet is the family's psychological state. Committing to the diet requires a great deal of faith. The parents (and grandparents) must believe that the diet can work. The diet is hard and sometimes takes patience. Although seizures often are reduced even during the admission week, that doesn't always happen, and the family needs to give it time.

Parents who start out as doubters will focus on the inevitable initial difficulties of the diet instead of focusing on the decrease in seizures and the improved behavior of the child as the diet starts. Without faith, it will be too frustrating when the child accidentally gets an incorrectly prepared meal, when she is irritable and demanding, or when he gets sick and has a seizure 3 weeks into the treatment. It will be too hard on the family if the child cries for afternoon cookies or Sunday night pizza.

If parents start out thinking positively, saying, "We will do whatever is necessary to give this diet a chance to work, the sacrifice is worthwhile if our child has a chance to become seizure free," then they are already halfway there. As stated earlier in this book, more than half of children will have fewer seizures and/or less medicine on the diet. The question will become whether the improvement is sufficient to continue the diet. Families will have a greater chance of success if they think of the opportunity to try the diet as a gift to the child, not as a punishment for having seizures.

Sometimes problems with the diet may not come from the parents or the child. They may come from a "How-will-my- grandchild-knowit's- me-if-I-don't-bring- Hershey's-Kisses?" grandma, or from a jealous "How-come-Peter- gets-all-the-attention?" sister. The optimism and faith that will carry a family through the diet (pardon us if this sounds a bit preachy) has to come from a team effort, encompassing the whole family, especially the child.

If the diet is effective and the seizures are under better control, if the child is functioning better, it becomes much easier to maintain the momentum. At the start it can be very tough. It is the willingness of the parents to meet the challenge that will carry the family through.

> *At first you are going to be afraid of temptation. You're going to feel bad about your child seeing others eat food he can't have. You'll be worried about what the diet's emotional effects will be. And you're going to be worried about whether your kid will cooperate. But you can live through it!*
>
> *If you have other kids, they can eat other foods. Try to be positive. The main thing to remember is, if the diet works your kid will be so happy to feel well again!*
>
> *I really have to thank you so much for putting me on the ketogenic diet back in 1991. I know that before I went on the ketogenic diet to help my seizures, I was on a lot of medication. The medication really did not help my seizures and made me have behavior and learning problems. If it was not for you, I don't think I would have made it this far in life. I am not sick anymore with seizures and I can concentrate and focus on my schoolwork. I am in college, sleeping away during the week and doing great. I am so grateful to have had you as my doctor. Once again, thank you so much.*

GETTING THE CHILD'S COOPERATION

The diet is more likely to go more smoothly if children are enlisted—rather than ordered—to participate. Children do not like having seizures. They do not like being different from their friends. Often, the thing they hate most is taking medications. They want to be cured of their seizures. If possible, explain to a child, in an age-appropriate fashion, how the diet may help fix these problems. If parents communicate their own enthusiasm for the diet as something worth trying, something that really might work, most children will buy in. They will feed on your enthusiasm. Let brothers and sisters participate as well in this—they can be great motivators. We have seen a sister create a coloring book with the story of the diet admission to keep the child with seizures entertained. So don't start the diet if you and your child are not enthusiastic about trying it—without that enthusiasm, it will be too hard.

But no one should make promises that cannot be kept! Parents cannot guarantee to the child that the seizures will disappear completely or that there will be no more medication. These are goals, but they cannot be promises.

Sticking to the diet will ultimately be the child's responsibility. Parents can help by giving children the psychological and emotional power to handle the tough parts. Role-playing may be useful. Parents can try rehearsing what to say in difficult situations. For instance, a parent might pretend to be a teacher offering a cracker at snack time, and let a child practice saying, "That's not on my diet, thank you!" Or a parent might pretend to be a friend trying to swap a sandwich for the child's cheesecake at lunch and teach the child responses such as, "No, I'm on a magic diet. I have to eat my own food." Children on the diet usually exhibit amazing self-control and willpower. They often handle the diet far better than their parents do—especially when they are doing well.

An example is Sarah, who had a stroke at birth and was 5 years old when she first came to Hopkins. Her one-sided seizures were hard to control, and she was a candidate for surgery. Before undergoing brain surgery, however, her family decided to try the ketogenic diet. Sarah did very well, and her seizures were better for a time, but ultimately she did not have good enough seizure control. Surgery was scheduled. Sarah would say, "What I dream about is having french fries again when I'm not on the diet anymore." So the night before surgery a nurse brought Sarah french fries. Sarah's response was "I can't have these. I'm still on my special diet."

Older children who try the ketogenic diet often need someone on whom they can vent their anger and frustrations. It is far better if this can be someone other than his or her parents. For teens and preteens, it may help to set up special telephone (or email or texting) times when they can talk to someone, perhaps a counselor or a mentor who has already been through the diet. This may start with a weekly call and then gradually become less frequent. Through these calls children can report successes and discuss problems, receive reinforcement, and hear stories about others who went through the same thing.

One of our counselor's favorite lines, when things seem particularly bleak and a child wants to quit the diet, is "Hey, it's up to you. No one is making you stay on the diet. You are always free to choose to stop the diet, to go back to having seizures. It's all up to you." Giving the responsibility to the child eliminates the parents and counselor as bad guys and empowers the child to see the reality that if the diet is indeed working, the choices are really very simple.

> *When Michael began to moan for a cookie I told him, "Michael, the epilepsy is your problem, and you have to solve it. We are here to help you, but most of the work is going to be yours. You're a big guy, you can handle it."*

Update: Michael stuck with the diet and now has been off it for several years. He still has a rare seizure, but he does well in school and is a first rate basketball player.

During the admission week we also try to have our new parents speak to some parents who have either had their child on the diet for a while (or were on it in the past). This is very helpful in terms of a pep talk, although no medical advice is given. Some families will also communicate with their "roommates" long after the admission week. There's nothing like peer support!

SPECIAL EQUIPMENT

The essential pieces of equipment for the ketogenic diet are a gram scale and a kit to test ketones in the urine. The urine ketostix are also important for the modified Atkins diet. The rest of the items listed in this section are things that other parents have found helpful.

Gram scales

The gram scale is the main calculating tool for the diet, so it is extremely important. Parents must either buy a gram scale or make sure that the hospital plans to supply one for the family to take home. Providing this service ensures that all parents get an accurate scale while saving them the time and effort of searching for one on their own. The scale should be accurate, should display weights in one-tenth gram increments, and should be portable.

Scales can be obtained through office supply or kitchen supply stores. Electronic digital scales, although slightly more expensive, are more accurate to the gram than manual scales. Examples of suitable scales include the Pelouse electronic postal scale and the Ohaus portable electronic postal scale.

Testing for urinary ketones

Strips for testing ketone levels in the urine are commonly available in drugstores, often combined with glucose tests used by diabetic patients (made by Bayer™ and available over the counter). These can be generic (e.g., Walgreens, CVS, Walmart) as well, and those are probably cheaper. A box of 50 ketostix should cost no more than $15 in the United States. Children on the ketogenic diet test urine periodically with these ketostix, usually daily the first week or two, then more sporadically.

Testing for blood in the urine

Parents are instructed to test the urine weekly for blood, which may be an early sign of kidney stones, one of the fairly common side effects of the diet. Hemoglobin (blood) in the urine may be tested using Bayer Multistix 10SG, which tests for several things, including hemoglobin and ketones. Because these strips are expensive, we recommend using them only once each week. A positive test for hemoglobin does *not* necessarily mean there is blood in the urine. The test should be repeated on several different specimens and then confirmed by a physician before a parent should become concerned.

Optional equipment that may be useful

Parents have found a variety of equipment helpful while their children are on the ketogenic diet. The following is a list gathered from many parents. It is meant as a source of ideas. All of this equipment is optional. Parents may buy these supplies if and as needed:

- Large collection of small plastic storage containers
- Bendable straws for drinking every drop
- Sippy cups for smaller children
- Screw-top plastic beverage containers
- Small rubber spatulas to be used as plate cleaners
- 1-, 2-, 4-, and 6-ounce plastic cups
- Measuring cup marked with milliliters or a graduated cylinder for weighing and measuring
- 10-cc syringe
- Pyrex custard dishes for microwave cooking and freezing meals
- Popsicle molds
- 6-inch nonstick skillet for sautéing individual portions with easy cleanup
- Travel cooler and/or insulated bag (useful to take home keto shakes, from hospital)
- One or two small thermoses for school and travel

- Toothpicks for picking up morsels of food to make eating fun
- Blender
- Milkshake wand or small hand beater
- Portable dual-burner electric camping stove for trips
- Masking tape for labels
- Microwave oven

To repeat, it is not necessary to own a lot of equipment before starting the diet. This list simply contains suggestions from various parents. Parents will gain more insight as to what equipment they will need as well as specific brands of food that are acceptable during their in-hospital ketogenic diet education. The only supplies that are absolutely necessary before starting the diet are a scale that measures in grams (to weigh foods) and strips for testing ketone levels in urine, which may be purchased or obtained from the hospital.

SPECIAL FOODS

Heavy whipping cream

THE ONLY ESSENTIAL FOOD RESEARCH parents need to do before starting the diet is to find out whether their neighborhood heavy whipping cream supply is 36% fat, 40% fat, or somewhere in between. The fat content of heavy whipping cream varies from one location to another, but most heavy cream is 36% fat.

The content of available cream will affect the calculation of the diet, so it is important to find what is available in a given neighborhood and to tell the dietitian before the child's diet is calculated. Make sure that there is no sugar added!

If you have any doubts about the content of your local cream, call the dairy directly. Dairies are required by law to know the fat percentage of the cream they supply. Remember, labeling laws do not require companies to list anything less than 1 gram of carbohydrate, protein, or fat, although fractional grams can affect the ketogenic diet! Once you find an acceptable brand, stick with it. Some local dairies will help to ensure that your local store stocks large containers of heavy whipping cream. Call your local dairy if you have any questions. We are indebted to Wawa dairies in the mid-Atlantic area, as they have provided heavy whipping cream free-of-charge for several years to families of children on the ketogenic diet. If you live in an area that has Wawa dairies, make sure to let your dietitian know.

OTHER FOODS AND FLAVORINGS

Many parents use flavorings to make the diet more fun for kids. These include the following:

- Baking chocolate

- Fruit-flavored sugar-free, caffeine-free diet soda or waters
- Pure flavoring extracts, such as vanilla, almond, lemon, maple, coconut, and chocolate. Make certain that they are pure, and check for alcohol content. Pure flavorings may be ordered from Bickford Flavorings (216-531-6006, or 1-800-283-8322)
- Sugar-free flavored gelatin such as Jell-O or Royal
- Nonstick spray such as Pam or Mazola No-stick for cooking
- Carbohydrate-free, calorie-free sweeteners. Saccharin (1/4 grain tablets of pure saccharin) is fine, despite some parents, concern about artificial sweeteners. In fact, these sweeteners are often very important to maintain a child's compliance and make foods more normal. Splenda and Stevia are also okay; liquid versions of these are probably best.

This list, like the equipment list, is intended as a source of ideas, not a must-buy-right-away order. The rest of the diet ingredients should be pure, fresh, simple foods: lean meat, fish, poultry, bacon, eggs, cheese, fruit, vegetables, butter, mayonnaise, and canola or olive oil.

READ THE LABEL! When using processed foods be sure to read the label carefully every times. Manufacturers often change the formulations of their products without prior notice. Therefore, each time you buy a processed food product, even if you have used it before, you must read the label very carefully. Remember that labeling laws do not require disclosure of contents less than 1 gram. Call the manufacturer if you have any questions.

BEWARE OF HIDDEN CARBOHYDRATES

Pay close attention to any foods or medicines that may contain carbohydrates. Nonsugar carbohydrates include mannitol, sorbitol, dextrin, and many ingredients ending in "-ose," such as maltose, lactose, fructose, glucose, sucrose, dextrose, or polycose®. All of these are carbohydrates and can possibly be broken down into glucose. They should be used sparingly when on the diet, and on the modified Atkins diet we calculate these "sugar alcohols" as part of the daily carbohydrate limit. Many foods, candies, and gums that are billed as "sugar-free" are NOT carbohydrate-free and cannot be used on the ketogenic diet. When in doubt, avoid it.

BARBARA AND MICHELLE: TWO CARBOHYDRATE SAGAS

Barbara had experienced no seizures in 6 months and was doing superbly well on the keto-

genic diet. In preparation for her follow-up EEG, the technician inadvertently gave her liquid chloral hydrate to allow her to sleep, but the oral chloral hydrate was in a carbohydrate base. The technician should have used carbohydrate-free chloral hydrate suppositories instead. It does not take much carbohydrate to quickly negate ketosis. Barbara's first seizure in 6 months occurred during that EEG.

Michelle lived in the city, but during the summer the family spent weekends at their beach house. She did well on the diet throughout the winter, with a marked decrease in seizure frequency. In the summer she again began having increased seizures, although only on weekends. The family would go to their summer house on Fridays. By Saturday Michelle's ketones would be low, and her seizures would increase. Her parents turned themselves inside out attempting to find the reason. They checked the foods and the environment, and they finally decided she must be allergic to the beach and their pool. They were about to sell the house.

At last, together with a nurse from Johns Hopkins, they again went over everything they did on Friday and Saturday. "When we arrived at the beach, we lathered Michelle with suntan lotion," they told the nurse. Aha! They checked the suntan lotion label: It was in a sorbitol base. Apparently enough sorbitol was absorbed through

Michelle's skin to affect her ketones and alter her seizure threshold! After switching to a sorbitol-free suntan lotion, the family continued taking Michelle to the beach with no recurrence of seizures.

Teenagers on the diet have reported that some lipsticks and soaps containing sorbitol may lead to seizures. Lowering ketosis through consumption of carbohydrates does not always cause breakthrough seizures, and often the children do fine without problems, but it can cause seizures. The good news is that when isolated breakthrough seizures occur, they nearly always can be eliminated again once the source is traced.

MEDICATIONS

Medications play an important role in the ultimate success of the ketogenic diet. Appendix A gets into more detail about this topic. Most children remain on medications (usually lowered doses or fewer medications, however) while on the diet. Starches and sugars are frequently used as fillers and taste enhancers in all forms of medication—particularly liquid medications. These starches and sugars can easily be overlooked in diet formulation, but they can impair a child's ability to maintain high levels of ketosis. Read the labels of all medications carefully. Take into account the carbohydrate content of all medications, whether routine medications taken daily or intermittent medications given to treat conditions such as a cold or an infection. When in doubt, ask your pharmacist. In general, tablets are better than liquids overall.

Ideally, the total carbohydrate content in medications should be less than 0.1 gram (or 100mg) for the entire day. Anything higher should be calculated into the meal plan's daily carbohydrate allotment. For example, a child taking 0.09 gram (90mg) of phenobarbital at bedtime in the form of three 0.03 gram (30mg) tablets receives 0.07 gram (72mg) of starch and lactose per tablet, or a daily total of 0.21 gram (216mg). There are carbohydrate-free forms of most of the older anticonvulsants. Some of the new anticonvulsants do not come in sugar-free or carbohydrate-free form. If they must be continued, the carbohydrate content can be calculated into the diet. In some instances, the sugar-free intravenous form of the medication can be used orally. During the starvation and diet initiation phase of the diet, the carbohydrate content of medications should be minimized by avoiding liquid preparations. The filler in pills may be ignored or calculated into the carbohydrates allotted. Pills can always be crushed and given in heavy whipping cream, ketogenic eggnog, or even unsweetened yogurt.

Difficulty in prescribing medications for a child on the ketogenic diet often arises from the fact that many common over-the-counter and prescription medications are not available in a sugar-free form. Many of those listed as "sugar-free" are appropriate for use in the diabetic population but not for children on the ketogenic diet because they contain starch or small amounts of other carbohydrates.

THE FOOD AND DRUG ADMINISTRATION does not require the listing of inactive ingredients such as sorbitol in the labeling of oral prescription drugs. Even when ingredients are listed, their precise amounts are often not found on the label.

Manufacturers are also frequently reluctant to release information about the amounts of particular ingredients in a medication, contending that this is proprietary information or that formulations change frequently. However, they can usually be persuaded to release the information if it is for treatment of a specific patient.

A pharmacist who is willing to get to know the ketogenic diet and the child and to work with the family for the duration of the diet can be a critical and valuable asset, helping to interpret labels and calling manufacturers if necessary. In this era of many generic seizure medications, we also recommend that you ask your pharmacist not to switch from one generic company to another if your child is doing well on one particular product. Although they don't have to do this by law, it's a good idea, and most pharmacists (if you ask nicely) will oblige. Ask your pharmacist or dietitian to double-check the contents of specific brands as formulas can change:

- Multivitamins: Mead Johnson's Poly-Vi-Sol™ (liquid or drops) with iron or Mead Johnson's Unicap-M™, Bugs Bunny sugar-free™
- Carbohydrate-free calcium: Rugby's calcium gluconate (600 to 650mg) or Calcimix™ (500mg), OsCal™
- Carbohydrate-free toothpaste: Tom's Natural, Arm & Hammer, Ultra Bright

Routine medications that are taken daily should come from a single company because ingredient concentrations vary among manufacturers. General rules for the use of medications, a selected list of medications that have been used by children on the diet, and contact information for pharmaceutical manufacturers can be found in Appendix A at the back of this book. Most medications can also be made in a carbohydrate-free form by a compounding pharmacy. You can ask a local one or order from H&B Pharmacy (201-997-2010).

GETTING READY FOR THE DIET: THE KETOGENIC DIET TEAM

A team effort is needed to keep each child and family on track and help them to get through the challenges of the initiation and fine-tuning period. The ketogenic diet team, or "ketoteam," at Johns Hopkins currently includes three physicians, a dietitian, our parent support group, a pharmacist, a social worker, and a nurse practitioner, who are all familiar with the diet. Each plays an important role in both initiating and maintaining the diet. This may not be the case at your ketogenic diet center and that may be perfectly fine, but at the very least, you need *both* a dietitian and neurologist to help you (not just one). The dietitian must allocate enough time not only to teach the diet while the family is in the hospital for diet initiation, but also to help the family with questions and dietary changes after discharge. Some medical centers also have a nurse or physician's assistant who can help the family through the many small crises that do not require medical attention.

If a center is going to start children on the diet, it must also be prepared to adjust the diet and work with the family through the fine-tuning period for at least several months after discharge. We estimate that an average family requires 30–40 telephone hours of dietary and illness counseling during the first year on the diet. Email time is almost impossible to calculate, but equally high. The child and family are, of course, essential partners in the ketoteam as well.

ADMISSION FOR THE START OF THE DIET

At Johns Hopkins we find that it is easier to admit four children simultaneously for initiation of the ketogenic diet than to do it one at a time. The advantage of admitting several patients at once is not only the efficiency of teaching the daily classes to multiple individuals, but also the support that families in the group can provide to each other as they go through the learning curve and the tribulations of diet initiation together. Without the group there is a tendency for each parent to feel that he or she is the only person in the whole world who is burdened with such an overwhelming task. Families in each group often stay in contact after hospital discharge and are often brought back to clinic for follow-up on the same day. Groups are usually admitted every month, which allows us to get one group off to a good start before the next one comes in.

An example of excess ketoacidosis was Robert, a frail 3 year old with very difficult to control "drop" spells. His mother was eager to get started on the diet, so she eliminated all starches and carbohydrates 3 days before coming to Hopkins.

The fasting was started, and the next morning Robert was admitted to the hospital. That night he vomited once and did not want to take his fluids. The next morning he was very sleepy. By that evening he had vomited twice and vomited his first keto shake. Blood tests showed that Robert was overly ketotic, and without enough fluids he was also somewhat dehydrated. Some fluids and a small amount of glucose put him back on track and allowed him to take the keto shake and progress to the diet.

Occasionally we will readmit children who had tried the diet elsewhere and had shown some promise that the diet was working. Parents would ask if we could make their child completely seizure free and felt we could fine-tune the diet more. We found that our success rate with these children was similar to those that we initially started on the diet, and there were several who did better with adjustments to the diet (and sometimes with a fast). There were many reasons for less-than-optimal results. We will evaluate these children on a case-by-case manner, and most children can achieve better control with minor adjustments by their dietitian (or neurologist), without the need for a readmission and fast. For this reason, we will sometimes see children on the diet at other programs for a one-time second opinion with their keto neurologist's consent, but rarely do they restart the diet.

CHAPTER EIGHT

Calculating the Ketogenic Diet

Calculating the ketogenic diet requires a combination of a full nutritional assessment and an understanding of the child's medical condition, mixed with experience and intuition. In each case, a child's individual needs must be taken into account. At Johns Hopkins, we meet as a group a week in advance of every ketogenic diet week and discuss each patient's needs (e.g., ratio, possibility of fasting, calories, medications, etc.). Because each child is different, this really helps guide management.

ESTIMATING CALORIC NEEDS

Calculating the caloric requirements of an individual child requires consideration of both the child's current and desirable weight as well as the patient's activity level. However, calculating the caloric needs of children going on the ketogenic diet should not be any different than calculating their needs if they were on a regular diet. The dietitian needs to look at history of weight and length gain over the years and evaluate the child's current eating habits and patterns before estimating their nutritional needs. A 3-day food record with the exact amounts of food eaten plus a growth chart or detailed weight history is essential in figuring out a child's caloric intake. We often match the ketogenic diet calories to the prior 3-day food record calories.

The ketogenic diet is generally based on the recommended daily allowance (RDA) of calories for a child's weight, but it can be modified to allow for such factors as the child's activity level and natural rate of metabolism. The goal of the diet is to provide optimal seizure control and maintain adequate nutrition for growth. When we make our initial estimates of a child's dietary needs, we begin by assessing the age, weight, height, health, activity status, and a current 3-day food record for each child. The ketogenic diet may be beneficial when a patient maintains their growth percentiles and doesn't gain weight or lose weight too rapidly.

Underweight children need to gain weight in order to have sufficient fat reserves to burn for ketosis between meals. Obese children may need to lose weight because if there is too much body fat, a child may have difficulty obtaining sufficient ketosis to control seizures. Severely handicapped children may be smaller in size and weight than average for their age. That is just the start; because a child's activity level is also an important determinant of caloric needs, a very active child may need more calories than a less active one. Profoundly handicapped children, who sometimes are very inactive, usually require fewer calories than an average child.

There is limited evidence that calorie restriction makes much of a difference in seizure control. Although this may be true in animals put on ketogenic diets, we don't always see that in children. In fact, on the modified Atkins diet, many children eat *more* calories than before they were treated! However, there are some children who seem to respond to cutting calories. Every child is different (see Table 8.1).

PROTEIN

Recommended daily protein allowances are calculated for average children of a given height and weight and an average activity level. The goal is to reach as close to the RDA for age of protein as possible. In adolescents it may be difficult to achieve the proper fat to carbohydrate ratio if 1 gram of protein per kilogram of bodyweight is given. In this case we may use as little as 0.75 grams of protein per kilogram. Growth is closely monitored every 3 to 6 months and is used as a guide of adequate nutrition. The evidence, however, suggests that the biggest impediment to growth is overketosis, rather than insufficient protein.

TABLE 8.1 Estimating Energy Requirements (EER)

RDA Age	Kcal/kg	Protein/kg
0–5 months	108	2.2
0.5–12 months	98	1.6
1–3 years	102	1.2
4–6	90	1.1

RDA Age	Kcal/kg	Protein/kg
7–10	70	1.0
Males:		
11–14	55	1.0
15–18	45	0.9
19–24	40	0.8
Females		
11–14	47	1.0
15–18	40	0.8
19–24	38	0.8

Note. EER (kcal/day)=Resting Energy Expenditure x Activity Factor x Stress Factor. Source: Recommended Dietary Allowances, 10th ed., National Academy of Sciences, National Academy Press, 1989.

FLUID ALLOTMENT

Anecdotally, in the past it was thought that a fluid restriction on the ketogenic diet may help with increased seizure control. This probably was due to concentration of the urine and, therefore, apparently higher levels of urine ketosis. Recent studies and years of evidence have determined that fluid restriction has no effect on seizure control. Therefore, we try and maintain as close as possible to 100% of fluid maintenance values. These numbers are based on the child's weight in kilograms and are more of a goal fluid volume than a restriction.

BODY WEIGHT	FLUID ALLOTMENT
1–10kg	100ml/kg
10–20kg	1000ml+50ml/kg for each kg >10kg
>20kg	1500ml+20ml/kg for each kg >20kg

Fluid intake should be individualized and increased with an increase in activity or a hot climate. Children in warmer countries may need more fluids than colder climates. Fluids are encouraged during illness. Monitor your child for signs and symptoms of dehydration like cracked lips, decreased urination, and a dry mouth.

JAMES: A CASE STUDY

The case of James illustrates the thought process of a dietitian evaluating an individual coming in for ketogenic diet initiation:

James is a 4-year and 7-months-old male with a history of infantile spasms (myoclonic seizures) and developmental delay. Seizure onset was at 12 months of age. Seizure frequency is 100–150 jerks/day.

CURRENT MEDICATIONS: Topamax® 75mg BID, Depakote® 375mg TID, Tranxene® 0.9mg daily. Supplements: Bugs Bunny multivitamin/mineral.

LABS: No current labs available.

FEEDING ABILITY: No impairment—James feeds himself—no problems with chewing, swallowing, etc. No history of pneumonia or aspiration.

James's mother reports his appetite to be poor and states that he is a "picky eater." James normally eats a great deal of starches (pasta, bread, etc.) as well as vegetables. He does not like meat very much. He eats three meals and two snacks daily. Food preferences were recorded. Activity is low to normal—James participates in physical therapy once a week and recess at school. His bowel movements are normal for the most part. No known food allergies or intolerances.

THREE-DAY FOOD RECALL: Average intake 1,290kcal, 42 gram protein, vitamin/mineral consumption adequate with the exception of calcium.

WT: 18.4kg (HEIGHT 111.8cm (40.5lbs) 44 inches)

WT FOR AGE: 50–75%

HT FOR AGE: 75–90%

WT FOR HT: 25–50%

James's growth pattern has been relatively normal—both height and weight were proportional following the 75% to 90% curve until 6 months ago. His mother said that James has been the same weight for 6 months now, despite an increase in height. She attributes his lack of weight gain to a decreased appetite since the addition of Topamax®.

PHYSICAL ASSESSMENT: No physical signs of deficiencies. James appears to be well nourished, although quite lean.

Assessment

James does not appear to be at nutritional risk at this point. Despite not gaining weight for 6 months, he is still 95% of his ideal weight, and weight has crossed only 1 percentile. He looks healthy and is consuming what is recommended for age for protein, macro- and micro-nutrients (with the exception of calcium intake of only 700mg). Caloric intake is obviously a bit too low as seen by the lack of weight gain and the fact that James is under his ideal body weight. It is reasonable to start him at his current caloric intake (and increase later if necessary) at a 4:1 ratio. We do not want him to lose weight, and the high ratio will allow us to provide the fat needed for ketosis via the diet.

Initial diet

1,300kcal, 4:1 ratio, 1,400cc total fluid daily. To be given in three equal meals and two snacks of 75kcal during the day.

KCAL: 1,300 (70.7kcal/kg body weight)

TOTAL PROTEIN: 24.5 gram

TOTAL CARBOHYDRATE: 8 gram
TOTAL FAT: 130 gram
TOTAL FLUID: 1,400cc (100% of estimated maintenance needs)

Parental, Neurologist, and Nutritionist Goals

1. Seizure control.
2. Maintaining current growth curve. Increasing kcal in small increments (5% to 10% of kcal every 2 to 4 weeks) should be sufficient to attain this goal provided that seizures are well controlled. James will probably not only have improvement of appetite, but hopefully of activity as well if his seizures can be controlled.
3. Maintaining optimal nutritional status (maintaining growth and overall nutritional status long term).
4. Weaning medications once the diet is fine-tuned satisfactorily.

Plan

1. Implement diet, educate parents.
2. Attain biochemical indices to check nutritional status (visceral protein status, anemias, electrolytes, hydration, renal function, etc.).
3. Discuss Topamax® wean with physicians after 1 month of the diet. Weaning this medication aggressively might help improve James's appetite.
4. Order multivitamin/mineral supplement that meets patient's recommended micronutrient needs 100%.

5. Continue to track height, weight, seizure control, etc., via phone/email/fax.
6. See James at 3-month follow-up visit.

Once judgments are made about ideal weight, ketogenic ratio, and liquid allotment, the ketogenic diet can be calculated.

GENERAL RULES FOR INITIAL KETOGENIC DIET CALCULATION

1. Decide on an optimal level of calories. This should be done using a thorough medical and nutritional history and the dietitian and physician's professional judgment. Variables such as the child's activity level, frame size, medical condition, recent weight gain or loss, and so forth, must be taken into account.
2. Set the desired ketogenic ratio. Most children ages 2–12 years old are started on a 4:1 ketogenic ratio. Medically compromised children may be started on a 3:1 ratio of fat to combined protein and carbohydrates. Children under 2 years of age and adolescents are usually started on a 3:1 ratio.
3. Fluid levels should be set at about 90–100% of maintenance for healthy, active children. Liquids are increased for fragile children and infants under 1 year of age.

4. Always strive to attain RDAs for protein (and never allow protein to fall below World Health Organization [WHO] standards).
5. The ketogenic diet must be supplemented *daily* with calcium, vitamin D, and a carbohydrate-free multivitamin with minerals. The diet is not nutritionally sufficient without supplementation.

Because this book is written for both parents and medical professionals, and because we believe that the diet works best with informed parents as part of the team, we believe it is important to know as much about the diet as possible. However,...

> THE KETOGENIC DIET should never be attempted without careful medical and nutritional supervision.

Roseanne is a girl who almost died because her parents started her on the ketogenic diet without consulting a doctor. She was 5 years old when she was admitted to Hopkins's intensive care unit with pneumonia, dehydration, and a very low pulse rate. There were major concerns about whether she would survive the night. She appeared wasted and fatigued and looked as though she had been starved by her parents.

The nurse called the child abuse team. The parents arrived a few minutes later, having fol-

lowed the ambulance from the referring hospital. They seemed very nice and very concerned. They said that Roseanne had suffered from lack of oxygen at birth and was quite developmentally delayed. At 5, she still could not sit by herself or communicate. Roseanne had experienced seizures since she was 6 months old and had been treated with many medications without much success. Her parents had come to the conclusion that not only were the medications not helping, but their side effects were part of the reason for Roseanne's lack of progress.

"All those doctors were doing was experimenting on our daughter," they said.

Then the parents had seen Jim Abrahams's TV movie about a diet for epilepsy that would "get you off the medications." When they called Hopkins, they were told that Hopkins would not be able to put Roseanne on the diet for 3 months. Her parents felt they couldn't wait that long, so they started the diet by themselves.

"It wasn't so hard at first," they said, and the seizures were better, until the last month when she just didn't seem to want to eat. Then she started throwing up and breathing funny. "I guess now you'll have to take her!" the parents said.

Roseanne had pneumonia but was also severely acidotic, malnourished, and dehydrated. With intensive care over the course of a week she gradually came around and was able to be dis-

charged home, but not on the diet. Until she had built up her reserves and had become better nourished, we felt that the diet posed too much of a risk. Frustration with the medical profession and impatience with the processes involved almost resulted in the child's death.

How a dietitian calculates the diet: Another example

1. **AGE AND WEIGHT.** Fill out the following information:

   Age _____

   Weight in kilograms _____

   Mary has been prescribed a 4:1 ketogenic diet. She is 4 years old and currently weighs 15 kilograms (33 pounds). Her dietitian has determined that this weight is appropriate for Mary.
2. **CALORIES PER KILOGRAM.** After a full medical and nutritional assessment, a dietitian will assign a calorie per kilogram level for diet initiation.

   The dietitian has set Mary's diet at 72kcal/kg. (Note that this figure involves a dietitian's judgment; it is usually based on comparing the child's current intake with the RDA.)
3. **TOTAL CALORIES.** Determine the total number of calories in the diet by multiplying the child's weight by the number of calories set per kilogram.

Mary, age 4 and weighing 15 kilograms, needs a total of 72x15 or 1,085 calories per day.

4. **DIETARY UNIT COMPOSITION.** Dietary units are the building blocks of the ketogenic diet. A 4:1 diet has dietary units made up of 4 grams of fat to each 1 gram of protein and 1 gram of carbohydrate. Because fat has 9 calories per gram (9x4=36), and protein and carbohydrate each have 4 calories per gram (4x1=4), a dietary unit at a 4:1 diet ratio has 36+4=40 calories. The caloric value and breakdown of dietary units vary with the ketogenic ratio:

RATIO	FAT CALORIES	CARBOHYDRATE PLUS PROTEIN CALORIES	CALORIES PER DIETARY UNIT
2:1	2gx9kcal/g=18	1gx4kcal/g=4	18+4=22
3:1	3gx9kcal/g=27	1gx4kcal/g=4	27+4=31
4:1	4gx9kcal/g=36	1gx4kcal/g=4	36+4=40
5:1	5gx9kcal/g=45	1gx4kcal/g=4	45+4=49

Mary's dietary units will be made up of 40 calories each because she is on a 4:1 ratio.

5. **DIETARY UNIT QUANTITY.** Divide the total calories allotted (Step 3) by the number of calories in each dietary unit (Step 4) to determine the number of dietary units to be allowed daily.

Each of Mary's dietary units on a 4:1 ratio contains 40 calories, and she is allowed a total of 1,085kcal/day, so she gets 1,085/40=27 dietary units per day.

6. **FAT ALLOWANCE.** Multiply the number of dietary units by the units of fat in the prescribed ketogenic ratio to determine the grams of fat permitted daily.

    On her 4:1 diet, with 27 dietary units/day, Mary will have 27x4, or 108 grams of fat per day.

7. **PROTEIN+CARBOHYDRATE ALLOWANCE.** Multiply the number of dietary units by the number of units of protein and carbohydrate in the prescribed ketogenic ratio, usually one, to determine the combined daily protein+carbohydrate allotment.

    On her 4:1 diet, Mary will have 27x1, or 27 grams of protein and carbohydrate per day.

8. **PROTEIN ALLOWANCE.** The dietitian will determine optimal protein levels as part of the nutritional assessment, taking into account such factors as age, growth, activity level, medical condition, etc.

    Mary's dietitian has determined that she needs 1.2 gram of protein per kilogram of body weight (18 grams total).

9. **CARBOHYDRATE ALLOWANCE.** Determine carbohydrate allowance by subtracting protein

from the total carbohydrate+protein allowance (Step 7 minus Step 8 above). Carbohydrates are the diet's filler and are always determined last.

Mary's carbohydrate allowance is 27–18=9 grams of carbohydrate daily.

10. **MEAL ORDER.** Divide the daily fat, protein, and carbohydrate allotments into the desired number of meals and snacks per day. The number of meals will be based on the child's dietary habits and nutritional needs. It is essential that the proper ratio of fat to protein+carbohydrate be maintained at each meal.

Mary's dietitian has decided to give her three meals and no snacks per day:

	DAILY	PER MEAL
Protein	18g	6g
Fat	108.0g	36.0g
Carbohydrate	9g	3.0g
Calories	1,085	361

Note: This example is simplified for teaching purposes. In reality, most 4 year olds would be prescribed one or two snacks in addition to their three meals. The snacks would be in the same ratio (4:1) and the meals reduced by the number of calories in each snack.

11. **LIQUIDS.** Multiply the child's desirable weight by the value shown on the chart listed earlier in this chapter to determine the daily allotment of liquid. Liquid intake should be spaced throughout the day. Liquids should be noncaloric, such as water, or decaffeinated zero-calorie diet drinks. In hot climates the

cream may be excluded from the fluid allowance (in other words, liquids may be increased by the volume of the cream in the diet). The liquid allotment may also be set equal to the number of calories in the diet.

Mary, who weighs 15kg, is allowed 1000+(50x5)=1250mlx.9=1125cc of fluid per day, including her allotted cream.

12. **DIETARY SUPPLEMENTS.** The ketogenic diet is deficient in some nutrients. Multivitamin and mineral supplements are required. In choosing a supplement it is important to consider carbohydrate content. Children who are not medically compromised can usually be adequately supplemented with an over-the-counter, reputable multivitamin and mineral supplement and a separate calcium supplement. Most children do well with commercially available supplements, although these have been alleged to lack some micronutrients.

CALCULATING MEAL PLANS

Calculating the meal plan, in contrast to the diet prescription, is a fairly straightforward procedure. There are currently two different ways of calculating the meal plans: by hand or by computer.

The hand calculation method uses exchange lists and rounded nutritional values for simplicity. This method is cumbersome, time-consuming, and based to a certain extent on nutritional averages. It is, however, the method that was used at Johns Hopkins and elsewhere with much success before the availability of personal computers. It is important that dietitians become familiar with the hand calculation method in order to fully understand the logic of meal planning, and in case a computer is not available in a pinch.

There are several computer programs available at many centers that are used by the dietitian to create meal plans. One such program is KetoCalculator (see Chapter 9). Because the computer program uses data about the precise nutritional content of specific foods, whereas the hand calculation method relies on averages in order to simplify the math, the computer program may result in slightly different numbers of calories and grams for a given meal than the hand calculation method.

> NO PROGRAM SHOULD be initiated or changed without the oversight of a dietitian to be certain that the nutritional information is up-to-date.

Generic Group A and B vegetables and fruits can be exchanged with both methods of meal calculation. It is easy for parents to switch from one Group A vegetable to another or one 10% fruit to another, depending on the child's whims or what is available in the grocery store. The exchange lists assume that there will be some variety in the diet. If the child only likes carrots and grapes—which contain the highest carbohydrate levels on the exchange lists—then she could end up with less than optimal seizure control. In this case the meal plans should be recalculated specifically for carrots and grapes.

The precision of the computer calculations shows the minor differences between the content of, say, broccoli and green beans. For most children these minor differences are of little importance. Therefore, once the computer has calculated a meal plan, and assuming that the child is doing well on the diet, exchanges may still be made among the foods on the fruit and vegetable exchange lists. If better seizure control is needed, however, in some cases it may be achieved through the use of specific meal plan calculations instead of exchange lists.

With the availability of the computer program, we no longer use meat exchange lists. The fat and carbohydrate contents of meats vary too greatly. The exchange lists are still used with hand calculations.

The dietitian provides parents with a set of basic meal plans before they go home from the hospital. When parents call the dietitian to discuss meal plans, they can refer to these basic meals by title. The basic meal plans are:

1. Meat/fish/poultry, fruit/vegetable, fat, cream
2. Cheese, fruit/vegetable, fat, cream
3. Egg, fruit/vegetable, fat, cream

The meat and cheese should be designated specifically (i.e., chicken, fish, parmesan) in actual meal plans. When specifics are added, the result will probably be a basic set of six or eight meal plans sent home from the hospital with the parents.

AVERAGE FOOD VALUES FOR HAND CALCULATIONS

	Grams	Protein	Carb	Fat
36% Cream	100	2.0	3	36
Ground beef	100	23	—	16
Chicken	100	31.1	—	3.5
Tuna in water	100	26.8	—	3
10% Fruit	100	1.0	10.0	—
Group B vegetable	100	2.0	7.0	—
Fat	100	—	—	74
Egg	100	12.0	—	12
Cheese	100	30.0	—	35.3
Cream cheese	100	6.7	3.3	35
Peanut butter	100	26.0	22	50

Note: A food contents reference book, such as Bowes & Church's Food Values, is helpful for current information on specific foods. As discussed in Chapter 5, the fat content of heavy cream should be consistent (e.g., 36%), and butter should come in solid, stick form, not whipped or low calorie.

CROSS MULTIPLICATION: THE KEY TO USING THE FOOD LIST

Question: If 100 gram of 36% cream contains 3.0 gram carbohydrate, how much cream contains 2.4 gram of carbohydrate?

Answer: 80 gram of 36% cream contains 2.4 gram of carbohydrate.

Sample calculation

1. Jeremy, a 9-year and 3-month-old boy, is to be placed on a 4:1 ketogenic diet. His actual weight is 32kg, and his height is 134cm. According to the standard charts, he is at 50% for height but 90% for weight. His ideal weight is estimated at 29kg.
2. The dietitian estimated Jeremy's calorie allotment at 60 calories per kilogram. One of the dietitian's goals was to have Jeremy gradually achieve his ideal weight. Toward this end, Jeremy's total calorie allotment is set by multiplying his ideal weight by 60:29x60=1,740 calories per day.
3. Each of Jeremy's dietary units will consist of:

   4 gram fat (9 calories per gram)=36 calories

   1 gram carbohydrate+protein (4 calories per gram)=4 calories

   Total calories per dietary unit=40 calories

4. Jeremy's dietary units will be determined by dividing his total daily calorie allotment (Step 2) by the calories in each dietary unit: 1,740 calories/40 calories per dietary unit=43.5 dietary units per day.
5. Jeremy's daily fat allowance is determined by multiplying his dietary units (Step 4

above) by the fat component in his diet ratio (4 in a 4:1 ratio): 43.5x4=174 gram fat.

6. Jeremy's protein needs are at a minimum 1 gram of protein per kilogram of body weight. His ideal weight is 29kg, so he needs at least 29.0 gram protein daily.
7. Jeremy's daily carbohydrate allotment is determined by multiplying his dietary units (Step 4 above) by the 1 in his 4:1 ratio, then subtracting his necessary protein (Step 6 above) from the total: 43.5-29=14.5 gram carbohydrate per day.

Jeremy's complete diet order will read as follows:

	PER DAY	PER MEAL
Protein	29.0g	9.7g
Fat	174.0g	58.0g
Carbohydrate	14.5g	4.8g
Calories	1,740	580

Note: Most children are now given a meal plan that includes one or two snacks, which would diminish the quantity of food in the three main meals. If Jeremy does not lose weight, is not in sufficient ketosis, or turns out to not be as active as originally thought, the caloric amounts will be recalculated during the fine-tuning period.

CALCULATING A MEAL	JEREMY'S TUNA SALAD
1. Calculate the whipping cream first. Heavy whipping cream should take up no more than half of the carbohydrate allotment in a meal.	1. Jeremy is allowed a total of 4.8 grams carbohydrate per meal. To use half of this carbohydrate allotment as cream, calculate the amount of 36% cream that contains 2.4 grams of carbohydrate. (See note on cross-multiplication.) Jeremy should eat 80 grams of 36% cream, which contains 2.4 grams of carbohydrate.

CALCULATING A MEAL	JEREMY'S TUNA SALAD
2. Calculate the rest of the carbohydrates (fruit or vegetables) by subtracting the carbohydrate contained in the cream from the total carbohydrate allotment.	2. For his remaining 2.4 grams of carbohydrate, Jeremy can eat 35 grams of Group B vegetables, or twice as many Group A vegetables.
3. Calculate the remaining protein (chicken, cheese, or egg) by subtracting the protein in the cream and vegetables from the total protein allowance. The total amount of protein may occasionally be off by 0.1 gram (over or under) without adverse effect.	3. The 34.3 grams Group B vegetables and 80 grams 36% cream contain a total of 2.3 gram protein (0.68+1.6=2.3). Jeremy is allowed 9.7 grams protein per meal, so he can eat as much tuna as contains 9.7−2.3=7.4 grams protein. Referring to the food values chart, this works out to be 28 grams tuna.
4. Calculate the amount of fat to be allowed in the meal by subtracting the fat in the cream and protein from the total fat allowance.	4. Jeremy has to eat 58 grams fat with each meal. The cream and tuna contain 29.3 gram fat, leaving 28.7 grams of fat to be mixed in with his tuna fish. Jeremy will get 39 gram mayonnaise, which contains 28.9 grams fat. (Note that mayonnaise actually has fewer grams of fat than oil does and also contains some protein and carbohydrate. The hand calculation method does not account for these variations).

CALCULATING MEAL PLAN

	Weight	Protein	Fat	Carbohydrate
Tuna	28g	7.4g	0.5g	—
Group B vegetable	33g	0.7g	—	2.3g
Fat	39g	—	28.9g	—
36% cream	80g	1.6g	28.8g	2.4g
Actual total	9.7g	58.2g	4.7g	

	Weight	Protein	Fat	Carbohydrate
Should be	9.7g	58.0g	4.8g	

The 4:1 ketogenic ratio of this menu may be double-checked by adding the grams of protein+carbohydrate in the meal and multiplying by 4. The result should be the amount of fat in the meal, in this case 58 grams. Since (9.7+4.8)x4=58, the ratio is correct.

NOTES ON JEREMY'S LUNCH

- Jeremy likes his cream frozen in an ice cream ball (slightly whipped), flavored with vanilla and saccharin, and sprinkled with a little cinnamon.
- Jeremy's mom arranges the vegetables in thin-sliced crescents or shoestring sticks around the tuna.
- If Jeremy doesn't like as much mayonnaise with his tuna, some of his fat allowance in the form of oil can be calculated and whipped into the cream one hour after it goes into the freezer. The fats on the exchange list can be used interchangeably—a meal's fat can be provided as all mayonnaise, half mayonnaise and half butter, or the oil may be calculated and mixed with the butter, depending on the child's taste and what makes food sense. In the case of hiding fat in ice cream, oil works nicely because it is liquid and has little flavor.

SOME COMMON QUESTIONS AND ANSWERS

Q. *How do you add extra ingredients to a meal plan when calculating by hand?*

A. Take the tuna salad as an example. Suppose Jeremy wants to sprinkle baking chocolate shavings on his ice cream and bacon bits on the tuna salad. You would add a line for bacon and a line for baking chocolate in your hand or computer calculation. Then choose a small quantity, perhaps 5 grams of bacon and 2 grams of baking chocolate, and fill in the values for protein, fat, and carbohydrate of each. The quantities of other ingredients would then have to be juggled downward until all the columns add up to the proper totals. Bacon, which contains protein and fat, will take away from the meal's tuna and mayonnaise allotment. Baking chocolate, which is primarily fat and carbohydrate with a little protein, will take away from the amount of tomatoes in the meal. As the overall carbohydrate allotment is very small and the nutritive value of chocolate is less than that of vegetables, no more than 2 grams of chocolate should be used in a meal on the 4:1 ratio. With the accompanying computer program, an additional ingredient may simply be filled in on a blank line and the other ingredients adjusted until the actual totals match the correctly prescribed ones.

Q. *When is it necessary to make calorie adjustments?*

A. Weight should be monitored on a weekly basis for the first month, and height on a monthly basis. Infants should be weighed and measured accurately at the pediatrician's office about every

2 weeks. At least during the first 3 months, the ketogenic diet team should be informed monthly of a child's height and weight changes and any other relevant information. Once a child is started on the diet, changes in the diet order are usually made in response to the child's own performance—weight loss or gain, growth in height, seizure control, and so forth. We evaluate in this manner and may make adjustments based on these factors throughout her time on the diet.

Q. *How often should a child eat on the ketogenic diet?*

A. The number of meals and snacks included in a child's diet should approximate her pre-diet eating habits (when possible), the family's schedule, and always take into account her nutritional needs. Infants will need to be given about six bottle feedings a day. Toddlers will probably need three meals and one or two snacks. Older children might need three meals and only one snack. Some children gain better ketosis overnight and achieve early morning seizure control by having a bedtime snack. Snacks are sometimes used to test how many extra calories are needed for a child who is losing weight and whether the extra calories cause any seizure activity problems.

Sarah was doing well on the diet, eating three meals and one afternoon snack. Her seizures were virtually gone during the day, but she was still having seizures early every morning. At her follow-up checkup the dietitian learned that Sarah was eating dinner at about 5:30P.M., going to bed around 7:30, and waking up at 7:00 for breakfast. It seemed that in the 13.5 hours between dinner and breakfast, Sarah was running out of fats to make ketones! The dietitian offered the family the choice of having Sarah eating dinner later, or of having an evening snack. They decided on the snack. Once Sarah started eating her snack at bedtime, the early morning seizures disappeared.

Q. *Is it necessary to use half of the carbohydrate allotment as cream?*

A. Using up to half of the carbohydrate allotment as cream is a guideline, not a hard and fast rule. It's meant to replace milk for children who drink milk, and cream can be an easy way to fit a lot of fat into the diet in a way that most children enjoy. However, children who do not like milk do not have to drink the cream; they will just have to have more mayonnaise, butter, or oil. Some children like to eat fat, some don't. Some children love cream, some don't. As long as the diet makes food sense, there is no need to use half of the carbohydrate allotment as cream.

A DIET ORDER TEST

Lily is 24 months old and weighs 12 kilos. She is 86.5cm. tall. Both her height and weight are at the 50th percentile. She is going to start on a 4:1 ketogenic diet. What will her diet order read?

1. At age 2 years, Lily's calorie per kilogram requirement will be approximately 75 calories per kilogram. (As indicated previously, calorie requirements vary with the metabolism and activity level of the child and must be individually assessed.) Her ideal weight is the same as her actual weight, 12 kilograms. So Lily's total calorie allotment is 75x12=900 calories per day.
2. Lily's dietary units will consist of 40 calories each, the standard for a 4:1 diet.
3. Lily's dietary units are determined by dividing her total calorie allotment by the calories in each dietary unit. So she will have 900/40=22.5 dietary units per day.
4. Lily's daily fat allowance is determined by multiplying her dietary units (22.5) by the fat component in her ratio (4 in a 4:1 ratio). She will thus be allowed 22.5x4=90 gram fat per day.
5. Lily's protein and carbohydrate allotment is 22.5 grams per day, determined by multiply-

ing her dietary units (22.5) by the 1 in her 4:1 ratio. As a young, growing child she may need 1.1–1.5 grams of protein/kg. Her weight is 12kg, so allowing 1.2 grams of protein per kilogram per day makes her protein allotment 14.4 grams per day.

6. Lily's daily carbohydrate allotment is determined by subtracting her protein allotment (14.4 grams) from the total protein and 1 carbohydrate allowance (22.5 grams): 22.5–14.4=8.1 grams carbohydrate per day.

Lily's complete diet order will read as follows:

	PER DAY	PER MEAL
Protein	14.4g	4.8g
Fat	90.0g	30.0g
Carbohydrate	8.1g	2.7g
Calories	900	300

Note: As mentioned previously, most 2 year olds eat one or two snacks in addition to their three meals a day. This example has been simplified for teaching purposes.

A MEAL TEST

For dinner, Lily would like to eat grilled chicken with fruit salad and a vanilla popsicle. How would you calculate this meal?

1. Start from the per-meal diet order. Lily is allowed a total of 2.7 grams carbohydrate per meal. To use half of this allotment as 36% cream, her popsicle should contain 45

grams cream, which will provide 1.35 grams carbohydrate.

2. To provide her remaining 1.35 grams carbohydrate, she can have 13g of 10% fruit.
3. The 10% fruit and 36% cream contain a total of 1.03 grams protein. Lily's total protein allotment for the meal is 4.8 grams, so she can eat as much grilled chicken as will provide 4.8−1.03=3.77 grams protein. This works out to 12 grams chicken.
4. Lily is allowed 30 grams of fat in each meal. The chicken and cream contain a total of 16.5 grams fat. Lily should eat 17g of butter or mayonnaise to provide the additional 13.5 grams fat allotment.

Lily's dinner plan will read as follows:

CHICKEN CUTLET WITH FRUIT SALAD

	Weight	Protein	Fat	Carbohydrate	Calories
36% Cream	45g	0.9g	16.2g	1.4g	155
Chicken Breast	12g	3.7g	0.3g	—	18
10% Fruit Exchange	13g	0.1g	—	1.3g	6
Butter	17g	0.1g	13.8g	—	125
Actual total		4.8g	30.3g	2.7g	304
Should be		4.8g	30.0g	2.7g	300

Notes on Lily's meal: The chicken can be pounded to be very thin to make it look bigger on the plate. The fruit salad will be pretty if composed of small chunks of water-packed canned peaches and fresh strawberries. Lily thinks it is fun to pick up the chunks with a toothpick. The cream can be diluted with some allotted water, sweetened with saccharin, flavored with four or five drops of vanilla and frozen in a popsicle mold in advance of the meal. Lily loves butter; she will eat it straight or it can be spread over her chicken. A small leaf of lettuce can be added to the meal for extra crunch.

LIQUID FORMULAS

The consistency of the ketogenic diet can be modified for all children, with various diets prior to admission. It can be calculated for bottle-fed infants, small children making the transition from bottle to soft food, or children with special feeding problems. The ketogenic diet can be formulated in any texture—liquid, soft, solid, or a combination—and can be easily used even by children who need to be fed by nasogastric or gastrostomy tube. Multiple studies stress how easy, well-tolerated, and beneficial it can be to use the ketogenic diet as a formula-only treatment.

As discussed previously, seizures or the side effects of anticonvulsant medications may affect a child's ability to eat properly. If the seizures are controlled or medications can be reduced while on the ketogenic diet, the child may be able to work with different therapists to transition from a soft diet to a diet with more textures. The process of calculating the diet and of establishing calorie levels and the grams of fat, protein, and carbohydrate permitted on the ketogenic diet is the same regardless of the consistency of the food.

There are many options for using formula for the ketogenic diet. Based on the formula that the child is on prior to diet initiation, a comparable keto formula is chosen. The formula can consist of three components mixed together with water to equal the correct calorie and ratio or KetoCal®, manufactured by Nutricia North America, which comes as a ready-to-feed liquid (in "tetra-paks") or as a powder. The KetoCal® Liquid comes in a 4:1 ratio, is nutritionally complete for children over 1 year of age, vanilla flavored, contains fiber, has no trans fats, and has only 15% saturated fats. KetoCal® powder is formulated in either a 3:1 or 4:1 version and is nutritionally complete for children over 1 year of age. All KetoCal® products are milk based and can be taken orally or via enteral feedings. There is also a new formula called KetoVolve® that is not on the market at time of publication but is manufactured by Solace Nutrition. This formula will have no trans fats, is 100% whey protein versus casein/whey mixture, and is lactose free. The company also states that it will be kosher and halal certified.

The Modular formula consists of three parts:

1. Ross Carbohydrate-free (RCF)®
   —Soy-based protein, avoids symptoms of cow's milk sensitivities
   —Available through Abbott in a concentrated liquid: 13 fluid ounce cans; 12 per case
2. Microlipid® (Mead Johnson)®
   —A safflower-oil emulsion that mixes easily in solution
   —Available in 89ml bottles; 48 bottles per case
3. Polycose® Powder (Abbott)®
   —Source of calories derived solely from carbohydrate
   —Available through Abbott in powder form (350 gram cans); 6 per case

In the case of multiple food allergies or stomach intolerances to intact proteins, there is another formula that can be used in the modular formula instead of RCF®.

4. Complete Amino Acid Mix®
   —Essential and nonessential amino acids
   —Indicated for patients with milk protein allergy
   —Needs complete vitamin supplementation
   —From SHS-Nutricia

Carbohydrate-free multivitamins and minerals, calcium supplements, and sterile water are added to complete the mixture.

FOOD VALUES FOR LIQUID DIET CALCULATION

	Quantity	Kcals	Protein	Fat	Carbohy-drate
RCF® con-centrate	100cc	81kcals	4.0g	7.2g	—
Microlipid®	100cc	450kcals	—	50.0g	—
Canola Oil	100g	827kcals	—	93g	—
Polycose® powder	100g	380kcals	—	—	94.0g
Complete Amino Acid Mix®	100g	328kcals	82g	—	—

Because it is emulsified, Microlipid® mixes easily with the other ingredients compared to oil. However, Microlipid® can be more expensive than corn oil or canola oil. Vegetable oil (e.g., canola) may be used for larger (older) children or when expense is a factor. MCT oil may also be added to a formula if the dietitian thinks it is needed, for instance, to loosen stools or boost ketosis. (More details on MCT oil in Chapter 20.)

TO SET UP A LIQUID MEAL PLAN

Emily was a 13-month-old girl admitted for the ketogenic diet in an attempt to achieve better control of her intractable seizures that had continued despite heavy medications. She had been fed by gastrostomy tube since she was 8 months old. She was started on a 3:1 ratio at 80/kg and protein at 1.6/kg of desirable body weight.

Emily's age: 13 months
Length: 29.7 inches (76cm), 50th percentile for age
Weight: 26.4lbs (12kg), 95th percentile for age
Weight/length: 98th percentile
Calories/kg: 80
Protein requirement: 1.6 grams, per kg
Ketogenic ratio: 3:1

Using the above numbers in the formula described earlier in this chapter, we calculate the diet order via the following steps (note: numbers are rounded to 0.1 grams.)

1. Calories: 80 (kcal/kg)x12 (kg ideal weight)=960 calories per day
2. Dietary unit: 980 (kcal)/31(kcal/dietary unit)=31.6 units per day
3. Fat allowance: 3 (as in 3:1)x31.6 (dietary units)=94.8 grams, fat
4. Protein: 1.6 (grams, per kg ideal weight)x12=19.2 grams, protein
5. Carbohydrate: 31.6 (protein 1 carbohydrate)−19.2 (protein)=12.4 gram carbohydrate

Emily's daily diet order follows. This will be divided into the number of meals or bottles she regularly gets in a 24-hour period.

Daily: Protein 19.2 grams, fat 94.8 grams, carbohydrate 12.4 grams, calories 960

Ketogenic diet for Emily using a *modular formula:*

1. Calculate the amount of RCF® needed to satisfy the child's protein requirement by cross-multiplying.

   Emily is 12kg. Emily's protein requirement is 1.6 grams per kilogram of desirable body weight, or 1.6x12=19.2 grams per day. 100cc of RCF® formula contains 4.0 grams of protein. Emily will need 480cc RCF® concentrate to meet her 19.2 grams protein requirement.

2. Calculate the fat in RCF® by cross-multiplying, and calculate enough Microlipid® to make up the difference.

   100ml RCF® contains 7.2 grams fat. Emily's 480cc of RCF® contains 34.5 grams. Subtract the 34.5 grams fat from the total 94.8 grams fat needed (94.8-34.5=60.3 grams). Remaining fat is 60.3 grams.

3. To calculate the Microlipid® needed to make up the remaining 60.3 grams fat in Emily's diet, cross-multiply. There are 50 grams of fat in 100ml Microlipid®=Emily will need 120.6ml Microlipid®

4. Calculate an amount of Polycose® powder sufficient to meet Emily's carbohydrate requirement.

5. The liquid allotment is set at 90cc per kilogram, giving Emily 1100cc liquid per day.

	Quantity	Protein	Fat	Carbohydrate
RCF® concentrate	480cc	19.2g	34.5g	—
Microlipid®	121cc	—	60.3	—
Polycose® powder	5g	—	—	4.7g
Sterile water	500cc	—	—	—
Total	100cc	19.2g	95g	4.7g

Emily's RCF® and Microlipid® total 601cc (480cc RCF®+121cc Microlipid®). Her water allotment will therefore be 1100-601=499cc. This will be rounded to 500cc.

EMILY'S DAILY FORMULA

Note: In practice this meal would be rounded to the nearest gram for convenience in measuring.

PREPARATION OF KETOGENIC LIQUIDFORMULA

1. Measure the RCF® concentrate and Microlipid® separately in a graduated cylinder.
2. Weigh the Polycose® powder on a gram scale and blend with above ingredients.
3. Add sterile water, reserving 10–15cc per feeding to flush the tube. Shake or stir.

4. Divide into the number of equal feedings the child will receive in a 24-hour period and refrigerate, or refrigerate full amount and divide into individual portions at feeding time.
5. Bring to room temperature or warm slightly before feeding.
6. Remember to supplement this formula with vitamins and minerals.

Samuel is a 9-month-old male with infantile spasms. He is on Enfamil 20 calories per ounce, drinking about 4–5 ounces every 3–4 hours, including overnight bottle feeds. On average, per the parents' report, Samuel is taking in 30 ounces per day. Samuel was admitted to start the ketogenic diet to reduce his spasms.

	Quantity	Protein	Fat	Carbohydrate
KetoCal® 4:1	100g	15g	72g	3g
KetoCal® 3:1	100g	15.3g	67.7g	7.2g
Ketocal® 4:1 Liquid	100ml	3.09g	14.8g	1.73g

Weight: 8.1kg (17.8 pounds) 5–10th percentile
Length: 70cm (27.5 inches) 20th percentile
Weight/length: 25%

Samuel will be started on a 3:1 ratio and using KetoCal® 3:1. His average intake of calories was 600 per day, which provides him with 75 calories per kilogram. The dietitian makes the decision to continue with the same calorie amount.

To prepare this formula using KetoCal®:

Because Samuel is on a 3:1 ratio, we will use KetoCal® 3:1. There are 699 calories per 100 grams of KetoCal® 3:1. Because Samuel needs 600 calories, divide that number by 6.99.

Samuel's daily formula using KetoCal®

86 gram of KetoCal® 3:1, 815cc of water

Parents should continue giving Samuel 4–5 ounces every 3–4 hours. Once Samuel starts to gain some feeding abilities, we will work with speech therapy and feeding therapy on starting some baby food and oils.

Liquid feedings may be given orally or through a tube. They may be given by continuous feeds or as periodic bolus feedings. The tubes may be flushed with sterile water as needed. It may be beneficial to continue the exact same feeding regimen that the child was on prior to initiating the diet.

Children on liquid feedings who do not have a swallowing difficulty, such as growing babies, may be transitioned to soft foods by gradually substituting the equivalent soft foods for a portion of their bottle feedings.

The liquid ketogenic formula is relatively expensive. However, because the liquid ketogenic diet is considered a therapy rather than a food, a family can try and have their insurance or WIC cover the cost. There is a sample letter at the back of the book that can help you.

CHAPTER NINE

KetoCalculator

This chapter was written by Beth Zupec-Kania, RD, from The Charlie Foundation.

Computer technology is valuable in assisting with the management of diet therapies for epilepsy. Keto-Calculator is a unique program that computes and stores diet information (see Figure 9.1). It was designed to calculate diets quickly whether you are in the middle of preparing a meal or are creating a series of new meals. The program is available online (www.ketocalculator.com), which makes it readily accessible wherever there is Internet access.

KetoCalculator may be used to create variations of the ketogenic diet. It has the flexibility to calculate the Ketogenic Diet ratios (5:1, 4:1, 3:1, 2:1) as well as the MCT oil diet, modified Atkins, and the LGIT (approximately 1:1). The program may be used to design diets for any age group and can be modified to the specific dietary needs of an individual. KetoCalculator can be utilized to create meals with baby foods, solid foods, liquid diets (formulas), or any combination of these.

The advantage to using an Internet-based system is that the food database is updated regularly. The database includes several hundred foods. The U.S. Department of Agriculture's Food Composition

Database is the main source of macronutrient data for natural occurring foods. Commercial food product information is obtained directly from the manufacturer. The carbohydrate content of medications and supplements is also obtained directly from the manufacturers.

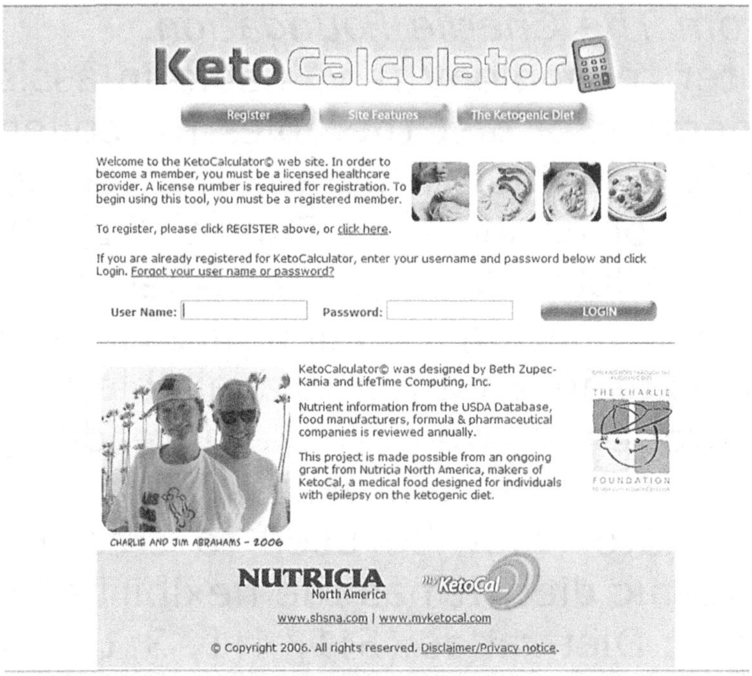

FIGURE 9.1

[Screenshot of www.ketocalculator.com.]

KetoCalculator is intended for use by people who are under the supervision of a health care team, and some features of the program are only viewable to these professionals. The program is free to health care providers who are then able to grant access to families. Health care providers may register for the program via the Web site (www.ketocalculator.com) . Once registered, a username and password are provided as well as instructions for navigating the program. The providers can then grant access to caregivers by creating a separate username and password. Access to the program is secure, and caregivers are only able to view their diet (and not the diets of other people). The following features are available through the caregiver access:

Create and Display Meals
Weekly Menu Planner
Handouts
Create and Display Snacks
Fluid and Diet Schedule

The menus that are provided in the program display gram weights of food that are specific to the Classic Ketogenic Diet and the MCT Oil Diet. These values may be converted to household measure for liberal diets, as shown in the table at the end of this chapter.

DIET CALCULATION

Prior to creating meals or snacks, the dietitian must enter a *Diet Calculation.* The diet calculation is tailored to the needs of the each individual and should be adjusted during the course of therapy by the dietitian. The *Diet Calculation* includes a calorie level, the ratio of the diet, and the appropriate amount of protein to provide the recommended dietary allowance (RDA) for the individual based on their weight and age. A sample *Diet Calculation* is shown in Table 9.1.

Once the diet calculation has been created, the total protein, carbohydrate, and fat are equally divided into the number of meals that are to be consumed daily. Three meals a day is the most typical diet plan, however, this can be tailored to the needs of the individual. For example, a 1-year-old may consume four meals daily.

TABLE 9.1 KetoCalculator Diet Calculation Screen

Diet date	2/23/2010		Daily	Per Meal
Age range	1-3	Fat	96.77	32.26
Desirable weight	15kg	Protein	18	6
Recommended calorie range	1000-1125	Carb	14.26	4.75
Daily calories	1000	Dietary units	32.26	10.75
Diet ratio	3:1			
Feeding route	Oral			
Meals per day	3			

CREATE AND DISPLAY MEALS

After the *Diet Calculation* is complete, the next step is to design meals.

The user may select from a list of Standard Meals. The Standard Meals are meals that are typical to the diet and consist of at least two foods that are high in fat, one high in protein, and one source of carbohydrate. The following list is a sample of the Standard Meals that are found in the program. Recipe instructions are included with certain meals.

Examples of Standard Meals

Breakfast sausage with fruit
Cheesecake
Chicken and spinach casserole
Chicken vegetable soup
Crabmeat salad with garlic dressing
Hot dog with vegetable
Lean meat with vegetable
Pork stir-fry
Scrambled eggs with avocado
Tuna salad with fruit

Once selected, the program automatically calculates the gram weight of each food in the meal; see Table 9.2.

This Standard Meal is created with the inclusion of two food groups. Group B vegetables are vegetables of similar carbohydrate content, and lean meat includes meat of similar protein and fat content. These food lists are assessable from the Handout link within KetoCalculator.

Meals may be individualized to suit preferences by changing the amounts of food using the up-down arrows. The user may also delete foods or add new foods to the meal. When these changes are made, the user must then manually correct the meal to match the recommended values shown at the bottom of the meal calculation.

TABLE 9.2

Example of a Standard Meal
Top of Form

Food Item	Grams		Fat	Pro	Carb	Calories	Units	Ratio
Cream, 36%	60	▲▼	21.6	1.2	1.8	206		
Group B vegetable	41	▲▼	0	0.82	2.87	15		
Lean meat (from list)	17	▲▼	2.84	3.96	0	41		
Butter	10	▲▼	8.11	0.09	0.01	73		
		Actual	32.55	6.07	4.68	335	10.75	3.0 3:1
		Recommended	32.26	6	4.75	333	10.75	3:1

The example in Table 9.3 illustrates the standard meal shown in Table 9.2 meal with the addition of a new food. In order to account for the avocado that has been added to this meal, a reduction in the cream and butter has been made. The vegetable and meat have also been adjusted.

A single meal may be edited in numerous ways to suit the preference of the individual. For example, if the user wanted to choose a specific meat and vegetable instead of using the choices in the Standard Meal, the meal could be easily adjusted by deleting those items then adding new foods. Once these new foods are selected, the meal can again be edited to meet the *recommended* values at the bottom of the calculation.

When a user edits a meal, the dietitian is notified to review and verify these edits. This notification occurs in the Main Menu of the dietitian's program. Once the dietitian has verified the meal, it becomes a printable meal. Without this verification, the meal cannot be printed. This is a cross-check system that helps to prevent the user from preparing meals that have not been reviewed. The printed version of the previous meal follows. Instructions may be added to the meals to clarify how the food items should be prepared.

TABLE 9.3

Example of a Standard Meal With Editing

Food Item	Grams		Fat	Protein	Carb	Calories	Units	Ratio
Cream, 36%	55	▲▼	19.8	1.1	1.65	189		
Group B vegetable	37	▲▼	0	0.74	2.59	13		
Lean meat (from list)	16	▲▼	2.67	3.73	0	39		
Butter	8	▲▼	6.49	0.07	0	59		
Avocado, California or Mexico (Hass)	20	▲▼	3.08	0.39	0.37	31		
		Actual	32.04	6.03	4.61	331	10.64	3.0 1:1
		Recommended	32.26	6	4.75	333	10.75	3:1

LEAN MEAT WITH VEGETABLE AND AVOCADO

Grams	
55	Cream, 36%
37	Group B Vegetable (from list)
16	Lean Meat (from list)
8	Butter

Grams	
20	Avocado, Hass

Instructions: Sauté sliced roast beef in butter in a small skillet until lightly browned. Pour remaining butter over warm vegetables. Serve cream as beverage or add diet caffeine-free root beer (free food). Serve sliced avocado with meat and vegetable.

CREATE AND DISPLAY SNACKS

In addition to meals, snacks can also be created in KetoCalculator. The calculation of a snack is similar to creating the calculation of the meals. It requires that the dietitian choose a calorie value and ratio. Standard snacks can be selected from a list of typical ketogenic snacks. They may also be modified to meet preferences. There are several innovative snacks recipes in this feature, which allows the user to test new items.

Table 9.4 is an example of a snack calculation for chocolate brownies. The recipe instructions (not shown) are provided with this snack. Once prepared, a brownie is cut to the gram weight identified to meet the desired calories and ratio.

The *actual* ratio of these brownies is 3.16:1, but this can be adjusted to a higher ratio, such as a 4:1, with the addition of fat, such as coconut oil or butter, into the snack calculation.

WEEKLY MENU PLANNER

After creating several meals and snacks, the user may plan a calendar of menus using the title of the meal or snack. The *Weekly Menu Planner* feature is helpful for organizing meals and snacks for upcoming days or weeks. This is especially helpful when there is more than one caregiver involved in managing the diet. First, the user selects a date from the calendar, then is prompted to select from the list of meals or snacks that were previously created and verified. A week of meals is illustrated in Table 9.5. The number that appears after the meal titles references the recipe for the meal.

TABLE 9.4

Example of Adjusting Fat to Brownies in KetoCalculator

Food Item	Grams		Fat	Protein	Carb	Calories	Units	Ratio
Chocolate Brownies	22	▲▼	10.01	2.09	1.08	103	3.17	
		Actual	10.01	2.09	1.08	103	3.17	3.16:1

TABLE 9.5 Week of Meals on the Ketogenic Diet

Meal	Sun February 8	Mon February 9	Tue February 10	Wed February 11	Thu February 12	Fri February 13	Sat February 14
AM meal	Keto pancakes – 5	Sausage/fruit – 17	Keto shake – 22	Cheesecake – 8	Quiche – 14	Keto shake – 22	Omelet – 11
Mid-day	Hot dog/celery – 3	Mac-N-cheese – 4	Cheese/veg – 9	Taco – 21	Tuna salad – 15	Turkey salad – 6	Chicken/veg – 26
PM meal	Spaghetti – 16	Stir-fry – 13	Veg soup – 10	Beef/veg – 18	Chicken salad – 2	Pizza – 12	Pork/veg – 24

FLUID AND DIET SCHEDULE

Another feature that assists caregivers with organizing the diet is the Fluid and Diet Schedule. This tool is intended to plan a daily routine of meal and snack times, nutritional supplements, medications, and beverages. It calculates the amount of fluid that is recommended for good health. The user can adjust the schedule during diet therapy as needed. This schedule is also available in a special format for individuals who are receiving their nutrition in liquid formulation, such as bottle feeding or feeding tubes.

ADDITIONAL FEATURES

KetoCalculator also includes supportive features to assist health care providers in the management of diet therapies. These are only viewable through the health care access.

- Vitamin and mineral supplement database with micronutrient and carbohydrate content
- Medication database with carbohydrate content
- Help Line; a question and response field for help with Keto-Calculator

KetoCalculator was designed in 2002 and has since received weekly editing and additions to its database, as well as annual updates to maintain the integrity of its digital framework. Use of this program has grown each year and is currently accessed by medical centers in 35 countries with several thousand users worldwide. Nutricia North America has provided the server space for this dynamic tool and has assisted with maintenance. Without their support, this program would not have been possible. For further information, you can email Beth Zupec-Kania at ketokania@gmail.com

Gram conversion to household measure

5 grams=1 teaspoon (tsp)
15 grams=1 tablespoon (tbl)
30 grams=2 tablespoons
60 grams=1/4 cup
120 grams=1/2 cup
180 grams=3/4 cup
240 grams=1 cup

CHAPTER TEN

All Those Crazy Supplements!

One of the most important goals for parents starting the ketogenic diet is to reduce their child's medications. Parents are surprised when they start the diet that we write more prescriptions than when they came in! Nevertheless, most of these supplements are essential for maintaining the diet and are vitamins and minerals to keep their child safe.

A child on a regular diet should be able to meet all of their vitamin and mineral needs just from eating their foods. However, the ketogenic diet is very high in fat and very low in carbohydrates, essentially eliminating a huge component of a regular diet. Vitamins and minerals are found naturally in fruits, vegetables, and animal proteins. However, in the United States all grains are enriched with vitamins and minerals. Through eliminating pastas, cereals, and bread and limiting fruits and vegetables, you are eliminating essential vitamins and minerals. The Dietary Reference Intakes (DRIs) have been established and provide recommendations for both macro nutrients (carbohydrate, protein, and fat) and micro nutrients (vitamins and minerals). It is provided free of charge for pdf download at this Web site: http://

iom.edu/Reports/2006/Dietary-Reference-Intakes-Essential-Guide-Nutrient-Requirements.aspx

MULTIVITAMINS

It is essential for all children on the ketogenic diet to be supplemented with a complete pediatric multivitamin meeting all of the DRIs for their age. There are a couple of vitamins that are low in carbohydrates that can either be purchased over the counter at a local pharmacy or via the Internet.

Some of the common vitamins that we use are Sugar-free Scooby Doo vitamins® (Bayer), Kirkman's Children Hypoallergenic Multi Vitamin® (Kirkman), Nano VM® (Solace Nutrition) and Phlexy Vits®(Nutricia). In the United States, other commonly used preparations include Unicap M® (McNeil), Centrum® (Wyeth), and Bugs Bunny Sugar-free® (Bayer). In Europe, Multibionta® (Seven Seas) is also available as a liquid formulation. Most general complete multivitamins are still low in calcium, requiring additional calcium supplementation. Nano VM® and Phlexy Vits® are the only vitamins that usually do not need additional calcium. Nano VM® is typically ordered over the Internet (http://www.solacenutrition.com/products/nanovm/nanovm.html) and is available for ages 1–3 years and 4–6 years. Nano VM® and Phlexy Vits® are powdered supplements that can be mixed in with fluids or small amounts of calculated applesauce or keto yogurt. The other vitamins can be chewed, swallowed, or crushed with water to provide via gastrostomy tube.

Formula-fed babies and older kids getting formula through a gastrostomy tube might not need additional supplementation. Compare the vitamins and minerals in the formula for the amount being provided to the DRIs, and supplement only those vitamins that do not meet 100% of the child's daily needs.

CALCIUM AND VITAMIN D

A lot of epilepsy medications are associated with bone loss and calcium metabolism. Many studies have shown that common medications for epilepsy lead to significant reduction in bone mineral density. However, it is unclear if supplementing more calcium and vitamin D than is required will help with calcium absorption. On the ketogenic diet there are very few calcium sources through foods. The only dairy that is eaten is cheese, and it's limited. Therefore, adding a calcium and vitamin D supplement will ensure that your child is getting at least the DRIs for their age.

Calcium is essential for the structures of bone and teeth and is also involved in vascular and neuromuscular functions. It is the most abundant mineral found in the body. Calcium is found in dairy products, such as milk, yogurts, cheeses, and ice cream; green leafy vegetables, such as broccoli and kale; and calcium-enriched foods, such as orange juice. Despite dairy products being high in fat they still have protein and some carbohydrates in them, making them difficult to use for the ketogenic diet. Heavy cream, the fat skimmed off of milk, contains minimal calcium. Therefore, calcium supplementation is essential on the ketogenic diet. Recently, the Institute of Medicine came out with new calcium guidelines (see Table 10.1).

Some common calcium supplements that we use are found in most pharmacies or available for purchase on the Internet. For tablets that can be crushed or swallowed, we use Nature Made brand of either 500 or 600mg calcium plus vitamin D or Caltrate® from Wyeth. There is an oral suspension from Roxanne called Calcium Carbonate 1250mg for 5ml oral suspension, and there is a powdered supplement from Now Foods called Calcium Citrate powder that can be mixed into liquids.

Vitamin D (calciferol) is also involved in bone health and is not found naturally in many foods products. It is synthesized in the skin through sun exposure, and it aids in calcium and phosphorus absorption. Vitamin D can be found in fatty fish, fortified milk, and other fortified foods like breakfast cereals. The Institute of Medicine also came out with new guidelines for vitamin D intake. The range is 400–600 International Units (IU) per day, but a child should not exceed 2500–4000IU per day (see Table 10.2).

You can purchase vitamin D from Now Foods or Carlson, in doses ranging from 100IU to 1000–2000IU per day.

TABLE 10.1 Calcium Guidelines from the Institute of Medicine

Ages	Recommended Dietary Allowance (mg/day)	Upper Level Intake (mg/day)
1–3 years old	700	2500
4–8 years old	1000	2500
9–13 years old	1300	3000
14–18 years old	1300	3000

TABLE 10.2 Vitamin D Guidelines from the Institute of Medicine

Ages	Estimated Average Requirement (IU/day)	Recommended Dietary Allowance (IU/day)	Upper Level Intake (IU/day)
1–3 years old	400	600	2500
4–8 years old	400	600	3000
9–13 years old	400	600	4000
14–18 years old	400	600	4000

ORAL CITRATES

Due to recent studies based on known side effects on the diet, many centers are providing oral citrate supplements. At Johns Hopkins we prescribe a potassium citrate (Polycitra K®) to all of our patients starting the diet. Since supplementing each patient we have seen a significant reduction in the amount of kidney stones by nearly 7 times, as shown in a study by a Hopkins medical student, Ms. Melanie McNally, in 2009. Oral citrates work to alkalinize the urine and solubilize urine calcium. They increase the pH in the urine, which increases urinary citrate and essentially decreases the amount of kidney stones. Polycitra K® is a powder supplement that can be added to water, and it is recommended to drink a lot of fluid as well to prevent kidney stones. For most children we dose it 2mEq/kg/day, for a young child we may give 15mEq twice daily (half of a 30mEq packet), and for an older child 30mEq twice daily (a full packet twice daily). Other supplements, like Citra K® and sodium bicitrate are fine and can be substituted if the pharmacy doesn't have Polycitra K®.

MIRALAX AND GI MEDICATIONS

Constipation and gastrointestinal intolerances to the ketogenic diet are both common side effects while on the diet. There have not been any studies looking at beginning antireflux medications when starting the diet, however, a high fat diet can cause gastroesophageal reflux and may be helped by starting an antireflux medication.

Constipation is one of the common side effects of the ketogenic diet. It is a diet very low in fiber, fresh fruits, and vegetables, and sometimes fluids. There are ways to help with constipation through foods using oils, MCT oil, and avocados, adding some prunes to the meals, exercising, and drinking enough fluid. But when that doesn't work, Miralax® is usually the safest and most effective way to treat constipation. It is another powder that gets added to water, but this one has no flavor! Some families report benefits with using Georges Aloe Vera®, but there are no studies regarding its efficacy, and there it is not approved by the FDA.

CARNITINE

Carnitine is a compound synthesized by the amino acids lysine and methionine and required for fatty acid to be transported into the mitochondria during the breakdown of fats for the making of metabolic energy. The active form of carnitine that is needed is called L-carnitine. The body makes enough carnitine on its own to help turn fat into energy; however, some children on a high fat diet can either not make enough carnitine on their own or have issues transporting it across the cell.

There are some clinicians that start all children beginning the ketogenic diet with carnitine and some that test levels and only give carnitine if the levels are low. Symptoms of carnitine deficiency can be fatigue and lethargy. The consensus of multiple centers is to test the carnitine level before the diet is started and then check every 3–6 months while on the diet and only supplement if there is a deficiency. Carnitine is another pill or liquid to take on top of everything else and can be expensive, so we use it at Johns Hopkins only when necessary. Carnitor® is the brand name product, but generic works fine. It comes in 330mg capsules or 1000mg/10ml liquid.

MCT OIL

MCT oil is a medium chain triglyceride oil compared to the regular household oils that are long chain triglycerides. In the 1970s MCT oil was introduced as a modification to the classical ketogenic diet. MCT oil was thought to produce higher ketosis; it is absorbed better than long chain fats and is carried directly to the liver. Because MCT oil was thought to be more ketogenic, less fat is used compared to the classical ketogenic diet, allowing for more protein and carbohydrates on the diet. Originally MCT oil would provide 60% of total prescribed calories, but this caused gastrointestinal distress and was reduced to 30% of total energy with long chain fats providing the other 30% of energy. The first double blind study was conducted comparing classical ketogenic diet to the MCT oil diet, and it showed no difference in the two groups attaining 50–90% seizure reduction. There is more information about MCT oil in the MCT diet in Chapter 20.

Because MCT oil is not sold in the supermarket and needs to be obtained from the Internet or specialty health food stores, it is not a supplement that is usually started at the initiation of the diet. It may be started for a variety of reasons such as high cholesterol and triglycerides or to increase ketosis, and it can be started in various doses of 5 gram to 25 gram at each meal or per day.

Coconut oil is one of the only oils available in most supermarkets in the health food section that contains MCT oil; depending on how the oil is extracted it can be 80–100% MCT oil. Many families are choosing to use coconut oil instead of other oils due to the higher MCT content. It still contains saturated fats. Coconut oil can be used in replace of all oils and is very heat stable and good for cooking and frying.

OMEGA 3

Omega 3 fatty acid (alpha linolenic acid) is an essential fatty acid; the body does not make it by itself, and it has to be consumed through food, but it is still necessary for human health. You can find omega 3 in fish, such as sardines, tuna, and salmon; some plants; and nut oils. Omega 3 is a poly unsaturated fatty acid, and plays a vital role in brain function and normal growth and development, may reduce the risk of cardiac diseases, and is anti-inflammatory. The highest concentration of Omega 3 is found in the brain and is important for cognition, behavioral functions, and performance.

For children, the recommended range of Omega 3 is to have 0.6–1.2% of total fat intake be from polyunsaturated sources. Due to the fact that the ketogenic diet is very high in fats, making the right choices for foods and fat sources should provide more than adequate amount of Omega 3. There is no established amount of Omega 3 that is too much to consume in one day, but the FDA recommends that total dietary intake of Omega 3 fatty acids from fish not exceed 3 grams per day for adults. Therefore, there is no reason to supplement with Omega 3 or assume that your child is deficient in Omega 3 fatty acid. However, one of the forms of Omega 3 is an oil and can easily be added into the diet.

SELENIUM

Selenium is an antioxidant nutrient that is involved in the body's defense against oxidative stress. One of the side effects of not eating enough selenium is cardiomyopathy, which is a weakening of the heart muscle or a change in the structure of the heart muscle. Regular diets provide adequate selenium through foods; however, because the ketogenic diet is restrictive it might not provide enough. Foods that contain selenium are Brazil nuts, tuna, beef, chicken, turkey, and enriched grains. Because we supplement every child with a multivitamin on the ketogenic diet we rarely see a selenium deficiency; however, the clinician must look at the vitamin that is chosen to determine if there is enough selenium for that child, and if not, then an additional selenium supplement is added.

SUMMARY

To make the ketogenic diet work for your child it is imperative that you provide your child with all of the prescribed supplements. Sometimes it's very difficult to force your child to take another pill or drink the flavored water, or even use a syringe to get in all of these supplements. Your keto team will work with you to find a supplement that works best for your child, such as a crushed pill versus a powder, but sometimes there are no other forms and that extra supplement is what is preventing your child from kidney stones or another side effect of the diet. There are many Web sites and chat rooms that talk about additional supplementation for children with all types of chronic illness. Do not start anything new unless you speak to your keto team and discuss the pros and cons of that supplement.

SECTION III

Life on the Ketogenic Diet

CHAPTER ELEVEN

The Expert Consensus and You

In 2007, the Charlie Foundation gathered together its Scientific Advisory Board at the American Epilepsy Society meeting in San Diego. Jim Abrahams commented on how variable at times the ketogenic diet could be, both in terms of who should start but more importantly *how* to do it. Several members of the Board had been approached in years past by societies who wished to create guidelines based on scientific evidence only. However, as most studies of the diet were retrospective (reviewed data collected over the years versus formal *prospective* studies with set criteria for enrollment), the scientific evidence might be considered insufficient to make recommendations. We all had strong concerns that such an *evidence-based* guideline would be a setback to the diet rather than a move forward.

Therefore, the "expert consensus statement" was born—a way to combine scientific evidence with personal experience from ketogenic diet experts; a total of 26 international ketogenic diet experts (as judged by known experience and at least one peer-reviewed publication about the diet). One-quarter were dietitians and 42% were from outside the United

States. Each author was assigned a topic based on their own research or experience, and then all sections were collected and combined. In addition, a short survey was created and sent to all authors to vote on certain topics. It was published in 2009 in *Epilepsia* and was endorsed by the Child Neurology Society.

How does it help a parent or patient? Well, it's important to know what the group felt were absolutely critical things to know and do for the diet. If your center is not doing them, you might want to bring them up. It's also good to know where flexibility and variability were common so each center may do their own thing. You don't need to read the entire document (unless you want to!); this chapter will highlight several aspects of it for you.

KEY TABLES

The following tables are perhaps the most important for child neurologists considering referring a child for the ketogenic diet. They list the indications and contraindications to starting the diet. These are felt to be conditions in which the diet may work particularly well and children should be referred sooner rather than later.

EPILEPSY SYNDROMES and conditions in which the KD has been reported as particularly beneficial:

Probable Benefit (at least two publications)

Glucose transporter protein 1 (GLUT-1) deficiency
Pyruvate dehydrogenase deficiency (PDHD)
Myoclonic-astatic epilepsy (Doose syndrome)
Tuberous sclerosis complex
Rett syndrome
Severe myoclonic epilepsy of infancy (Dravet syndrome)
Infantile spasms
Children receiving only formula (infants or enterally fed patients)

Suggestion of Benefit (one case report or series)

Selected mitochondrial disorders
Glycogenosis type V
Landau-Kleffner syndrome
Lafora body disease
Subacute sclerosing panencephalitis (SSPE)

There are also conditions in which the diet should not be used. These are usually screened for in advance by neurologists and pediatricians.

Contraindications to the Use of the Ketogenic Diet

Absolute

Carnitine deficiency (primary)

Carnitine palmitoyltransferase (CPT) I or II deficiency

Carnitine translocase deficiency

β-oxidation defects

Medium-chain acyl dehydrogenase deficiency (MCAD)
Long-chain acyl dehydrogenase deficiency (LCAD)
Short-chain acyl dehydrogenase deficiency (SCAD)
Long-chain 3-hydroxyacyl-CoA deficiency
Medium-chain 3-hydroxyacyl-CoA deficiency.

Pyruvate carboxylase deficiency

Porphyria

Relative

Inability to maintain adequate nutrition

Surgical focus identified by neuroimaging and video-EEG monitoring

Parent or caregiver noncompliance

Most of the group felt the diet should be offered after two medications have been tried and failed, regardless of the cause of seizures. Interestingly, about half the group would *not* offer the diet to a child with a clear structural cause for seizures that surgery would potentially help. At our center, we will, but we do counsel families that the chances of seizure freedom are somewhat less than when seizures are due to other causes.

The following section covers things that should be done in advance of a ketogenic diet admission.

RECOMMENDATIONS FOR PRE-KETOGENIC DIET EVALUATION

Counseling

Discuss seizure reduction, medication, and cognitive expectations

Potential psychosocial barriers to the use of ketogenic diet

Review anticonvulsants and other medications for carbohydrate content

Recommend family read parent-oriented ketogenic diet information

Nutritional Evaluation

Baseline weight, height, and ideal weight for stature

Body mass index (BMI) when appropriate

Nutrition intake history: 3-day food record, food preferences, allergies, aversions, and intolerances

Establish diet formulation: infant, oral, enteral, or a combination

Decision on which diet to begin (MCT, classic, modified Atkins, or low glycemic index)

Calculation of calories, fluid, and ketogenic ratio (or percentage of MCT oil)

Establish nutritional supplementation products based on Dietary Reference Intake

Laboratory Evaluation

Complete blood count with platelets

Electrolytes to include serum bicarbonate, total protein, calcium, zinc, selenium, magnesium, and phosphate

Serum liver and kidney tests (including albumin, AST, ALT, blood urea nitrogen, creatinine)

Fasting lipid profile

Serum acylcarnitine profile

Urinalysis

Urine calcium and creatinine

Anticonvulsant drug levels (if applicable)

Urine organic acids

Serum amino acids

Ancillary Testing (optional)

Renal ultrasound and nephrology consultation (if a history of kidney stones)

EEG

MRI

Cerebrospinal fluid (CSF) (if no clear etiology has been identified)

EKG (echocardiogram) (if history of heart disease)

AREAS OF CERTAINTY

There were some aspects of the consensus statement that were unanimous and clear to the expert group. Parents should be counseled in advance and expectations covered. Baseline labs need to be obtained (see Appendix F) and all children supplemented with a multivitamin and calcium. Medications should be changed to carb-free forms and weaned after 1 month if the parent desires. Follow-up should be at least every 3 months for the first year on the diet, with more frequent visits probably helpful for infants. Most centers felt the *alternative* ketogenic diets had a role and could be used (see Section IV). Fasting and admissions for the diet, although advocated by many as helpful, were not always necessary and could be avoided. At each clinic visit the risks and benefits of the diet should be discussed, but the minimum duration is 3 months and maximum before considering stopping is (usually) 2 years.

AREAS OF FLEXIBILITY

There were just as many, if not more, areas of flexibility. Fasting (done by about half the centers) and admissions (done by 88% of centers) are at the discretion of the center. Which diet (LCT, MCT, MAD, or LGIT) is up to the center and the parent. Although there are data that 4:1 may be better than 3:1 at the start of the diet, the ratio, calories, and fluid content of the diet is at the judgment of the dietitian rather than set in stone. Many of the other supplements, including especially carnitine, were debated and also flexible.

CONCLUSIONS

This consensus statement was a step in the right direction for the ketogenic diet worldwide. It proved that 26 experts could come together and put together a useful document to help each other and new centers starting ketogenic diet centers. It also shows that a general protocol for the diet could be created, as there were many aspects that were agreed upon, often completely by the entire group. The statement also showed that there are many, many ways to provide the diet, and none are necessarily wrong. This is a big part of what's new in this edition of this book—the ketogenic diet is not "one way or the highway" for every child. We suspect the consensus statement will be revised in 5–10 years, and it will certainly be interesting to see trends in the voting especially on some of the controversial topics.

CHAPTER TWELVE

Fine-Tuning the Diet

Fine-tuning the ketogenic diet typically occurs during the first few months of beginning the diet. However, it can also occur after years have gone by as a way to make the diet more effective. This can be an important part of making the diet individualized for your child, be it changes in calories, ratios, fluid allotments, or other variables such as medication dosing. Most changes can be done by phone and email when necessary.

We encourage close communication with the ketoteam as the dietitian adjusts the various components of the diet—calories, liquids, fats, recipes, ketogenic ratios, and so forth—to achieve the best level of ketosis for optimal seizure control and the best meals for the child and the family. This support can be crucial as the family searches for the proper foods, learns to read and interpret labels, becomes accustomed to preparing the diet, and integrates it into their lifestyle. Myriad questions arise as a child's body becomes accustomed to the diet and as the meals are prepared. Support for fine-tuning is particularly necessary when seizure control improves initially but the family is hoping for even better seizure control or for the child to be on even less medication.

Initiating the diet means not only changing the foods that are consumed but also changing the parents' and family members' attitudes and expectations about food and mealtimes. This is particularly true for small children where the small number of calories calculated is over estimated at the start or just seems "too small" and is raised by the parent who does the cooking, with resultant weight gain for the child and lack of optimal seizure control. We often make changes based on a child's body mass index and hunger level—if a child is happier and healthier, they may be more compliant with the diet as well.

Sometimes a child refuses to eat the cream or becomes too constipated. Adjustments to the child's diet must then be made. It takes at least 2 weeks to see if a change is effective. Because only one change can be made at a time, it may take several months of fine-tuning to see how much benefit the diet will provide for that child.

The fine-tuning phase is often the most time consuming for the dietitian as the family develops confidence in the diet and the ability to make decisions for themselves. There is often a bit of trial and error by the dietitian to find the *right* diet for the child. Although usually we start with a 4:1 diet, lower ratios may be better for some. Similarly, too many (or too few) calories have been seen (in some children) to lead to higher seizure frequency.

The goals of fine-tuning are:

1. To reduce seizures to a minimum—optimally for a child to become free of seizures.
2. To reduce seizure medications to a minimum—eventually and optimally for a child to become free of anticonvulsant medications.

Each family is asked to make a 3-month commitment to attempting the diet in order to give allow the fine-tuning phase to work. We ask this even before the family comes into the hospital to initiate the fasting phase of the diet. Of our families, 83% remain on the diet for at least 3 months. Every family is told that they may discontinue the diet any time they wish after the 3-month trial. However, because the initiation of the diet is so very labor-intensive for both the family and ketogenic diet team, this investment of time, effort, and money is not worthwhile if the diet is not given a good trial.

Our data would suggest that if the diet is going to work, it will do so within that first 3 months. Some other research suggests that the first 3 months may be the most important with stricter diets (e.g., 4:1 vs. 3:1 and 10 grams/day vs. 20 grams/day with the modified Atkins diet) and more likely to lead to seizure control. In this regard, although the first few months may involve this fine-tuning, we often loosen up on our restrictiveness after that. This isn't always the case, though, and even some children who have been on the diet for decades require some "tweaking" of their diet here and there.

EXPECTATIONS

Fine-tuning does not always lead to total freedom from seizures. During the initiation of the ketogenic diet and afterward, it helps if a family's expectations are realistic so that they are not setting themselves up for disappointment. Virtually all families have watched the videotape from the Charlie Foundation before diet initiation. In this tape Charlie Abrahams came to Hopkins severely impaired by his seizures and medications and walked out of the hospital 4 days later cured. This impression of the speed in which the diet works is reinforced by the story of the child with uncontrollable seizures in the Meryl Streep film, *First Do No Harm.* That child was also flown to Johns Hopkins and sent home cured.

These stories are both based on truth, but they are not typical, and certainly not universal.

- Not everyone is cured by the ketogenic diet.
- Not all of those whose seizures are substantially helped by the diet find the correct calorie level and ketogenic ratio during their initial stay in the hospital.
- Not all children are able to come off medication and remain seizure free.

We spend a lot of time with families during the initiation week going over their personal goals. Every family has different goals. For most, it's fewer seizures. For others, the primary reason to start the diet is fewer medications. For nearly all, it's a brighter, more alert child! We may also look at the EEG over time to see if there is improvement. Think what *your* expectations are before you start—you may even want to write them down somewhere safe and look at them again in 6 months.

With careful fine-tuning, however, more than one-half of the children starting the ketogenic diet at Johns Hopkins derive sufficient benefit that they remain on the diet for more than 1 year. Even Charlie Abrahams required a fine-tuning period. Charlie didn't go home from the hospital in 4 days. He remained several extra days in the hospital, sick and vomiting, until it was determined that a virus was causing his nausea. Even after he had returned home, it took days for Charlie to feel well. After this initial difficult period, Charlie became seizure free and eventually medication free. Still, he was often reluctant to eat, and persuading him to finish each meal was a major daily struggle for his mother. Two years later, when coming off the diet, he again had several seizures and had to go back on a modified diet. Eventually, Charlie was able to come off the diet and off medications—and remain seizure free for years.

The lessons to be learned from Charlie's case are important. Charlie's experience with the diet was, and is, a spectacular success. But this success did not come easily. When obstacles arose, his parents refused to become disappointed and discouraged. They put in a lot of hard work, maintained a tough attitude, and made the diet work for Charlie.

The most important thing for a parent to remember during the fine-tuning period is this: *You can, and you will persevere!* If your child is doing well at the start of the diet, that's terrific. But most children do not immediately become seizure free. Many never become totally free of seizures; others do become virtually, or even totally, seizure free after weeks or months of careful fine-tuning.

Only after working carefully with the ketoteam for several months will you have enough information to decide if there is sufficient improvement in your child to continue with the diet.

If seizures are controlled for even a few days at the start, the diet is likely to work. Long-term control can likely be established with patient fine-tuning. We suspect that at the end of 2 days of fasting and the 2 days of gradual introduction of the ketogenic eggnog, a child's blood serum ketones may reach a peak, providing a temporarily high level of seizure control. Once a child is at home and eating meals again, serum ketones may not be as high, even though the urine is still 4+. Increasing the ketosis by fine-tuning the diet may help.

Breakthrough seizures do not necessarily mean that the diet has failed; further fine-tuning may be likely to be beneficial. If seizures are improved, less frequent, or less severe, it may be hoped that further improvement will be achieved as the diet is adjusted.

Some of the factors that may have to be adjusted during this fine-tuning period are calorie allotment and distribution, the ketogenic ratio, meal plans, meal frequency, liquid intake, and anticonvulsant medication levels.

THE IMPORTANCE OF SLEUTHING

To master the fine-tuning process, parents and the ketoteam become adept at tracing the cause of any problem that arises. It is also important not to make a change based on one bad day—the next day could be much better with no changes! We usually make diet changes if things are worsening over a week or more.

If a child is having problems on the diet, the parents and the rest of the diet team must become private eyes. It often takes a detective's spirit to locate the source of a problem and fix it. The most common cause of a problem with the diet is that the child is getting the wrong amount or the wrong balance of food and liquid. There could be many reasons why the amount or balance of food and liquid are off:

- Is there an opportunity for the child to eat extra food at school or while playing at a friend's house?
- Is the diet prescription correctly calculated? The caloric needs of a disabled child may be much lower than those of a nonhandicapped child of the same age and size.
- Are commercial foods being used? They often contain hidden carbohydrates.

- If commercial foods are used, are they the exact brands and items called for in the menu? For example, different brands of bologna may have different fillers and different carbohydrate contents.
- Check the label—has the manufacturer changed ingredients?
- If calculations were made by computer, are the database entries for the ingredients correct?
- Is the child sick with a common virus or bacterial infection? Infections may trigger seizures both in children on the diet and in those on medications. Wait until the infection is gone then reassess how the child is doing.
- Is everything being measured on a gram scale except free fluids? Sometimes, after the diet seems to be working well, parents become lax and measure foods by eye rather than by scale.
- Are vegetables being weighed cooked or raw as specified?
- Are the peaches packed in water, as they should be, rather than in glucose-containing syrup or fruit juice?
- Is there a soft-hearted grandparent in the picture who is encouraging the child to cheat "just a little"?

It is not possible to list every problem and solution in this book, but the principle to remember is *be a sleuth.* Think it through. Don't give up. Look for clues. Was there a change in the number or kind of seizures at a certain time of the day or week? Did the problems begin following a certain meal plan or a specific family event? Sometimes the best thing to do can be to wait. If nothing is found that caused the worsening of seizures, allow the natural history of epilepsy (ups and downs of seizures) to play to your advantage. Things could get better just with time rather than increasing a medication.

JESSICA CAME IN FOR A CHECKUP after a year on the diet, and she was doing great. She talked like a little adult, whereas before the diet she had difficulty making sentences at all because her mind was so full of medication and seizures. She was still having some seizures, though. What she told us was that her grandmother liked to give her candy even though the candy gave her seizures. She said she was going to change that, though. She was going to start saying, "I can't have any more candy, Grandma. I'm on a special diet and I have to stay on my diet because I don't like having seizures!" Jessica had to stay on the diet for longer than the usual period of time. She would probably have gotten off sooner if her grandmother hadn't cheated.

If a problem develops after good seizure control has been established, parents should examine every aspect of their child's food and liquid intake, play habits, pharmaceuticals, and time with babysitters and relatives. The dietitian should listen to a parent describing exactly how each meal is prepared. If the dietitian cannot solve the problem, the physician may need to get involved. With persistence you can most likely isolate the problem and correct it.

REMEMBER: Illness, ear infection, the flu, or urinary tract infection may cause breakthrough seizures. See if a child is sick, and if the cause of breakthrough seizures might be temporary illness, before changing the diet. Illness is the most common cause of breakthrough seizures.

MEASURING KETOSIS

The efficacy of fine-tuning is measured by a child's seizure control but also by her level of ketosis. The general goal of fine-tuning, then, is to get the brain into a state of ketosis adequate to obtain optimal seizure control. Although we don't know for sure that ketones matter for everyone, they seem to for some children. Looking at a seizure calendar and trying to correlate seizures and ketones can help your ketoteam see if your child is "ketone-sensitive." If that is the case, then changing the diet (if ketones are low) may be beneficial.

We teach parents to check ketones daily by using a urine dipstick. This is an easy, cost-effective method for monitoring the level of ketosis. The paper stick, when dipped in the child's urine, turns color depending on the amount of ketones in the urine. The ketogenic diet has traditionally been fine-tuned to maintain the child's urine at 3–4+ketones, which turn the stick a dark purple in color (80–160mmol).

For babies and young children who are not yet toilet-trained, urine is collected by placing cotton balls in the diaper. Once the child has urinated, the cotton balls can be squeezed onto a dipstick for testing. For older children on the diet, peeing on a dipstick becomes second nature. For older children that are not continent, you can use the cotton ball approach, or periodically use a urine collection bag, available in physician offices.

The weakness of urinary ketone testing is that it is actually ketones in the brain, not those in the urine, that influence seizure control. Ketones in the urine can seem lower if tested after a child drinks a large quantity of liquid. They may vary with the time of day. These ups and downs, however, may have only an indirect relation to seizure control.

Preliminary evidence using blood ketones suggests that once the blood ketone level rises to more than 2mmol, the urine ketone level becomes 4+. That is the highest level the dipsticks can measure. Seizure control however, appears far better when serum levels are greater than 4mmol, way beyond that 4+urine level. So, a urine ketone test of 4+is *necessary* to establish that the child has ketosis but *not sufficient* to indicate very good ketosis. Therefore, in *some* situations, blood ketones may be important. However, we don't usually recommend our parents go home with blood ketone meters in all cases. We see this as generally unnecessary sticking of children so don't do it often. We usually do check serum ketones with the rest of the blood work at clinic visits.

COMMON PROBLEMS AT THE STARTOF THE DIET

For the first 2 to 3 weeks after the hospital discharge, the child and the family will have had the chance to adapt to the diet as it was initially calculated. This is the time we start making the small changes we call fine-tuning that can often make a major difference in a child's level of seizure control. The most common areas to be explored for fine-tuning potential are the following:

- Caloric intake
- Carbohydrate intake
- Distribution of meals
- Misuse of free foods
- Menu preparation
- Illness
- Ketogenic ratio
- Fluid intake
- Processed food content
- Function or use of gram scales
- Food values used in calculations

FINE-TUNING MEAL PLANS

Usually each child is given several (about six) meal plans, calculated by the dietitian specifically for that child, before leaving the hospital at diet initiation. These meal plans will probably be in the form of "chicken (or meat, or egg), Group B vegetable (or 10% fruit), fat, cream." As the child adjusts to the diet, the meal plans themselves may need fine-tuning. Physical reasons, such as weight loss or weight gain, may necessitate revising the meal plans, or a child may refuse to eat a basic diet component such as cream.

As parents prepare the diet meal, they will learn from their child what works and what does not work for them. One child who loves chocolate cream popsicles, for instance, may want to eat chocolate cream popsicles at every lunch and dinner. Another child who leaves the hospital with six basic meal plans may grow tired of them after a period and want more variety.

Once parents get the hang of using their gram scales and making up specific menus, some want to devise their own menus or add little treats to the diet to increase the child's enjoyment of meals or ability to participate in family events. Adding or changing ingredients is limited only by the mathematical confines of the ketogenic ratio and by the child's protein requirement.

Children, on or off the diet, often will ask for the same meal over and over. Because the meals are nutritionally balanced, a child can eat the same meal for breakfast, lunch, and dinner and for many days in a row. It is often the parents who get tired of seeing the same thing on their child's plate and demand new meals.

Of course, fats, carbohydrates, and protein must be kept in proper balance, and enough protein must be supplied in the diet to support a child's physical development. Still, parents and dietitians can find ways to include treats for the children that are properly calculated into the diet. After all, the object of the ketogenic diet is to control seizures. Within the limits of this goal, the diet can be made as easy as possible for a child to live with.

Parents should carefully research any and all new foods they wish to introduce into the diet, especially commercially processed foods. Foods whose protein, fat, and carbohydrate content are not clearly labeled should be avoided. So-called diet foods or sugar-free foods such as chewing gum may contain carbohydrates that make them inappropriate for the diet or at least make it necessary that they be calculated in.

NO ADDITIONAL MEALS SHOULD BE CREATED by parents until fine-tuning has been accomplished. Adding "fancy foods" just adds to the difficulty of teasing out what is wrong when ketones are low.

TIPS FOR TEENS (FROM A TEEN)

1. When using lipstick, soap, or suntan lotion, check for any kind of sugar. One time, I used some soap that had sugar in it. I didn't know that at the time though. That night I had seizures from it.

2. When at social events such as Youth Group, Prom, a school party, etc., focus on the socialization part of it. If the food bugs you, mingle and talk with people who are not eating food at the time.

3. Listen to music that is inspirational to you. This should be a song that helps you know "I can do this! I'm not alone!" When I started the diet, my favorite song to listen to was "Hero" by Mariah Carey. It helped me sooooo much!

4. Remember that even if the kids in your class or classes are eating candy, you are getting better even if it is tough. I know this issue all too well! When I was in middle and high school, the teachers would give out candy for no reason at all, and I'd be totally bummed out. However, I knew I was getting better and that thought helped me a ton!

5. When asked why you don't have to eat the cafeteria food, just say something like: "I don't want to get sick!" You could even do a twist on that. Say someone says "Hey! You are sooooooooo lucky! You don't have to eat the lunch lady's food!" You could just smile and joke with them saying

something like: "The lunch lady's food is ok, but I'm getting better by not eating it."

"FREE" FOODS

There are no foods on the ketogenic diet that are actually "free," meaning available on an unlimited basis. What are often referred to as "free" foods are those that can be eaten occasionally in small quantities without being calculated into the daily ketogenic menu plans. Free foods include 25 grams of lettuce; one walnut, macadamia nut, or pecan; three filberts; or three ripe (black) olives. Most other foods, such as sugar-free Jell-O or any carbohydrate-based snack food, cannot be used at all without being calculated into the diet.

Any added foods outside of meal plans can make a difference in seizure control. Children who eat free foods every day may find that they affect seizure control. For children who continue to have seizures on the diet, free foods should be the first thing restricted during the fine-tuning process.

WHEN SHE CAME TO US, Jennifer was tied in a wheelchair. She was so impaired by her drop seizures and her medications that she couldn't stand. She was already on a low-protein diet because her liver had been damaged by medication. Five days after she started the initial fast and ketogenic diet she was running down the hall! Everybody was so excited. Back home, she didn't need naps anymore. Her anticonvulsants were stopped. She was doing well and not having any seizures. Then the seizures came back, a little bit at first, and of course we had to recheck everything. It turned out that Jennifer liked nuts. She was allowed two "free" nuts per day. But her mother had started giving her extra nuts, seven per day, because she was begging for them and they made her so happy. Some of the nuts had honey that wasn't highlighted on the label but was in the ingredients. When we went back to two nuts a day the seizures came back under control.

SPECIFIC FOODS

Initial menus for the diet are usually calculated using "generic" fruits and vegetables but designating specific meats and fats. The use of processed foods such as hot dogs and deli meats may cause a drop in urine ketones and result in a rise of seizures. The content of these foods is hard to assess. The labeling of their content is not exact. They are usually high in carbohydrates and sodium and relatively low in protein. Therefore, while fine-tuning the diet of a child with continued seizure activity, parents are requested to withhold processed foods for 1 month to see if this has an effect. Most of our children do fine with these foods (in fact, we have one child who ate nothing but hot dogs every day!), but if they are new and seizures have increased, be aware and let your dietitian know.

FATS

Not all fats are equal. A child who is having difficulty producing sufficient ketosis may need to have the type of fats in her diet adjusted. It may help to reduce or remove the less dense fats such as butter and mayonnaise and substitute canola, flaxseed, olive, or MCT oil (Table 12.1). Medium-chain triglyceride (MCT) oil is more efficiently metabolized, helping to produce a deeper ketosis. We use MCT oil for only a portion of the fat allowance, however, because when ingested in large quantities it often causes gastrointestinal disturbances such as diarrhea or vomiting.

TABLE 12.1 The Protein, Carbohydrate, Fat, and Calorie Content of "Fats" (kcal)

	Grams	Protein	Fat	Carb	Kcal
Butter	100	0.67	81.33	0.00	735
Margarine, stick corn oil	100	0.00	76.00	0.00	684
Mayonnaise, Hellmann's	100	1.43	80.00	0.70	729
Corn oil	100	0.00	97.14	0.00	874
Olive oil	100	0.00	96.43	0.00	868
Canola oil	100	0.00	90.00	0.00	810
Flaxseed oil	100	0.00	100.00	0.00	900
Peanut oil	100	0.00	96.43	0.00	868
MCT oil	100	0.00	92.67	0.00	834
Safflower oil	100	0.00	97.14	0.00	874

We suggest using as much as possible unsaturated oils that contain a high fat level per gram and little or no carbohydrate or protein. Flaxseed oil is a good, heart-healthy choice. When using MCT oil we begin with 5 grams per meal, or 15 total grams daily, for children who need to go into deeper ketosis. This may be increased slowly, as tolerated, until seizure control seems as good as possible with minimal side effects.

FREQUENCY OF MEALS AND SNACKS

Not only is the *quantity* (calories) and *quality* (ketogenic ratio and nutritional content) of food important, but also the *timing* of food intake can influence the success of the ketogenic diet.

An individual on a normal diet stores energy for short-term use as glycogen and fat. During periods between eating or during starvation, the body first burns carbohydrate from food recently eaten, then burns carbohydrate that it has stored as glycogen, and finally begins to burn fat. Burning fat, in the absence of carbohydrate, results in ketosis.

Children on the ketogenic diet have virtually no carbohydrate in their diet, and they consume few calories, so they have virtually no stores of glycogen. Therefore, they depend on fat for their energy.

A child who is at his desirable weight has very little stored fat and, therefore, is dependent upon the fats he eats at each meal. If too long a time passes between meals, the child may run out of fat to burn. His body will then burn some of its stored protein, but this will make his ketones decrease, and seizures may result. In this way, we'll give extra snacks here and there, especially at times of the day with more seizures (e.g., nighttime).

WILLIAM WAS A 3-YEAR-OLD who was doing very well on the diet. His seizures decreased dramatically, but his parents noticed that he continued to have a few seizures early in the morning, before he woke up. On close questioning the dietitian discovered that the family fed William at 5:00P.M. and put him to bed at 7P.M. He didn't get up until about 7:30A.M. William's ketones always measured very low in the morning, which the ketoteam interpreted as a sign that he needed to spread out his food intake. The early morning seizures disappeared after his dietitian calculated a late-night snack into William's diet.

Children usually have breakfast in the early morning and eat lunch around noon, but dinnertime is very variable. Some children are fed supper as early as 5:30P.M. and then go to bed at 7:30–8:00P.M. This means that they will not have eaten for 12 to 14 hours before their breakfast.

This makes little difference to a child on a normal diet who has plenty of energy reserves stored as glycogen and fat. But a child on the ketogenic diet may not have sufficient reserves to maintain ketosis overnight. If a child eats dinner later or has a snack at bedtime, the body is less likely to run out of ketones during the night. This may help to control early morning seizures.

COMMON PROBLEMS IN THE FIRST MONTHS ON THE DIET

Weight gain

The most common error in initiating the diet is the improper estimation of a child's caloric needs. For some children the initial estimate of calories and ratio is appropriate, or at least sufficient, and seizures are completely controlled on the diet as initially prescribed. For some children, however, overestimation of caloric needs means that while seizures decrease after the initiation process, they are not as well controlled as they could be.

Overestimation of calories takes place partly because the recommended daily allowances (RDAs) of calories on which diet calculations are based are for average children of a given height and weight, with an average level of activity. However, the ketogenic diet is often used with children whose motor or intellectual capabilities are impaired to the point that they burn far fewer calories than average, healthy children.

It is tempting to start small, profoundly handicapped children on calories that are geared to more active children of the same height and weight, as a dietitian will usually prefer to err on the high side than to underestimate calories. However, we often find that such children gain weight at this calorie level, and it becomes necessary to cut back. It may be preferable to take better account of the child's activity level when making the original calculations. Restricting calories for less active children will result in better ketosis and earlier improvement in seizure control. It is also psychologically easier for families to add calories or a snack to the diet than to reduce calories.

100 CALORIES PER DAY=1 pound per month

If a child has lost a pound in 1 month, calculation will reveal that approximately 100 calories should be added to the daily diet. With these additional calories, the child should gain back the lost pound in a month. Once the child's proper caloric intake is reached, the weight gain or loss will stop. Remember: No two children are identical. Basal metabolic rates differ from child to child, and activity levels can differ markedly. In each case, excessive weight gain or loss indicates that caloric intake must be adjusted.

If a child is losing too much weight, the calorie level should be increased in increments of approximately 100 calories at a time (even less in small infants). Enough time should pass between increments so that an evaluation can be made as to whether the child's weight has stabilized, whether seizure activity has occurred or increased, and whether hunger is under control. If it is determined that extra calories are needed, instead of recalculating all the meal plans, a snack calculated at the prescribed ratio of fat to carbohydrate and protein may be added to the diet (calculating calories and ratios was further explained in Chapter 8). Adding a ketogenic eggnog snack to the child's daily meal plan may be a convenient alternative to recalculating all the meals in the short term while adjustments to the diet are being made. Twelve grams of macadamia nuts, which equals 100 calories, also make a good snack (the macadamia nuts, naturally in a 3:1 ratio, are sometimes eaten with a calculated amount of butter to achieve a 4:1 ratio).

For average people it takes approximately 3,500 calories to gain a pound. If a child has gained a pound in 1 month, then 3,500 too many calories have been consumed. Dividing the calories by the number of days (31 in a typical month) reveals that the child has consumed approximately 100 extra calories each day. By recalculating the diet at about 100 fewer calories, the dietitian can stop the weight gain.

Hunger

Because the physical quantity of food on the diet (the bulk) is smaller than in a normal diet, many children will feel hungry during the first week or two of the diet until they adjust. This may be especially true of overweight children, who will have their diets calculated to include some weight loss. However, ketosis itself decreases the appetite, so children are much less likely to be hungry when consistently high levels of ketones are reached, usually within a week of starting the diet.

If a child initially complains of being hungry, try to determine which of the following are true:

- She is really hungry.
- She has not yet adapted to the smaller portion.
- She wants the pleasure and comfort of eating.

Sometimes it is not the child who is hungry at all, but rather the parents who feel pity for the child or guilt about the small portions and who project their feelings about the diet onto the child. Other times, in the complex emotional atmosphere of diet initiation, a child's cries of hunger are actually declarations of rebellion against the parents. In any case, most children will lose their feelings of hunger once they adjust to the food they are consuming and achieve consistently high ketosis.

We recommend that parents deal with hunger without trying to add extra calories to the diet, at least for the first few weeks. Tricks to modify hunger without increasing calories include:

- Drinking decaffeinated diet soda or seltzer instead of water for at least part of the liquid allotment
- Freezing drinks, such as diet orange soda mixed with cream, into popsicles
- Eating a leaf of lettuce twice a day with meals
- Making sure that foods, such as vegetables, are patted dry so that water is not part of the weight
- Recalculating the diet plan into four equal meals, or three meals and a snack, while maintaining a constant level of calories and the proper ketogenic ratio
- *Decreasing* calories slightly to raise ketosis and suppress hunger

THE HUNGER PARADOX Ketosis is an appetite suppressant. If reducing calories on the diet leads to better ketosis, it may decrease hunger as well. Therefore, children who are getting too many calories and gaining weight on the diet may feel hungrier than those who are getting fewer calories. Children who are hungry on their diet may have been given too much to eat! Therefore, *reducing calories may help to relieve hunger.*

Constipation

Constipation can become a problem because of the small volume of food, low fiber content, reduced fluid intake, and high concentration of fat in this diet. Constipation may cause stomach pains and discomfort. Fortunately, it does not have to be an obstacle to continuing the diet. Using Group A vegetables in meal plans can help increase the bulk and fiber in the diet a little bit. Also, two leaves of lettuce, or about one-half cup of chopped lettuce, are allowed each day as so-called free food.

Make sure that the child is receiving the proper amount of liquid. Increasing daily liquid levels by 100 to 150cc may help combat constipation.

If a child continues to have problems with constipation, laxatives, stool softeners, or enemas may help. Full-strength enemas should not be used regularly because they can affect the lining of the intestine. Small amounts of Miralax®, Colace® (1% solution or suppository), Milk of Magnesia, Epsom salts, or MCT oil calculated into the diet might be effective in maintaining bowel regularity and preventing constipation. Fleets enemas and aloe vera are also useful. All laxatives must be sugar-free.

NON-DIET PROBLEMS

Children who are on the diet become irritable and cry for many reasons just as other children do. It is not always due to the diet.

Celeste, age 2, had been home from the hospital 4 days when her father called the doctor. "My wife is exhausted from staying with Celeste in the hospital," he said. "Now Celeste won't eat anything. She's crying, she's sleepy, she's whining all the time. We can't live like this!" His voice cracked with exasperation. "I can't take this diet!"

"How many seizures was she having last week, before she went into the hospital?" the doctor asked.

"More than a hundred every day."

"How many did she have during the starvation?"

"About 10 a day."

"How many did she have yesterday at home?"

"One."

"Let's not give up the on diet so fast then," the doctor said. "Maybe there's a reason why she is so sleepy and irritable." On further investigation, it was discovered that Celeste had developed a fever, and her pediatrician diagnosed a urinary tract infection. Once this was treated, Celeste continued on the diet and did very well.

When problems appear in a child on the ketogenic diet, don't always assume that the diet is the cause of the problem. A child may be irritable from the hospital stay or from the difficulty of making such a radical adjustment in her life. She may rebel against the extra attention and pressure to which she is being exposed. She may be coming down with the flu or a cold. A cautious approach to fine-tuning over several weeks or months after the start of the diet will make it easier to remain on the diet.

Thirst

Thirst is not a common problem for children on the ketogenic diet because ketones also decrease thirst. However, it is important to watch the child's urine output, particularly in hot weather, because extra fluid may be needed. In general, we do not restrict fluid any longer, so this should not be a problem.

It seems to be important for many children to space the consumption of liquids throughout the day and not to give a thirsty child a big drink all at once, as this can sometimes cause breakthrough seizure activity and can also leave the child thirstier later on. Some parents give their child a regular dose of water or diet soda (with no caffeine) every 1 to 2 hours during the day. Other children seem to be able to drink larger amounts of liquid with no seizures.

In hot climates or during summer months, the cream in the diet need not be counted as part of the allotted liquid. In effect, this raises the liquid allowance by the quantity of the cream.

A child may become dehydrated if the fluid allowance is insufficient. Signs of dehydration include dry lips and skin, infrequent urination, sunken eyes, and lethargy. Most thirst problems, as well as problems of excessive acidosis, can be corrected by increasing fluid intake, usually in increments of 10 to 20cc/kg of body weight per day until the problem is corrected. The ketoteam can determine adequate fluid replacement levels and ongoing fluid requirements by monitoring a child's weight, urine quantity, specific gravity of the urine, and ketone levels.

CHANGING THE DIET'S KETOGENIC RATIO

Raising the diet's ratio (fat-to-[protein+carbohydrate]) increases the amount of fats consumed, with the goal of increasing ketosis and thereby resulting in better seizure control. If a child is continuing to have seizures, and if careful, thorough sleuthing has not revealed a cause, then raising the ketogenic ratio may be considered. We raise ratios in half-point increments, from 3:1 to 3.5:1, or 3.5:1 to 4:1. We rarely go higher than this.

Occasionally the ratio is decreased during the fine-tuning period if a child becomes anorexic and will not eat, if she remains too acidotic, if she is experiencing frequent illnesses, or if she is having digestive difficulties on the diet. Most older children start the diet on a 4:1 ratio. They are then adjusted downward slowly after their first year on the diet.

Overweight children are an exception to this rule. We frequently start them on a diet in 3:1 ratio with restricted calories to facilitate weight loss. As they lose weight, they burn their own body fat, and this produces high ketones for them. As they approach their desirable weight, overweight children have less of their own body fat to burn, so we may need to increase the ratio to maintain the same high level of ketones. Adolescents often need a 3:1 ratio to provide sufficient protein within their caloric restrictions. Very young children are also usually started on a 3:1 diet to allow more protein for their growth.

MEDICATION LEVELS

The fine-tuning period usually involves adjusting medication levels as well as food and other nonfood factors. Unless a child displays signs of overmedication, it is preferable to wait several weeks after initiation before beginning to taper any medications. Only one medication should be tapered at a time, and diet changes should not be made at the same time as medication changes.

It is not uncommon for one or even a few breakthrough seizures to occur 24 to 72 hours after each decrease in medication dose. Parents and physicians should not reintroduce the medication or take any other action unless the seizures continue for more than a week. If the increase in seizures continues for a week, reintroduction of the medication may be necessary. Benzodiazepines such as clonazepam are addictive, and their withdrawal commonly produces seizures. For this reason, their reduction must be done very gradually to minimize withdrawal symptoms. A compounding pharmacy may be useful in preparing the increasingly dilute, sugar-free solutions needed for the weaning process.

Reducing anticonvulsant medications is a secondary but important goal of the ketogenic diet. Some children on the diet are able to stop taking all anticonvulsant medications and never have to go on them again. The situation varies for each individual.

Don't be in too much of a hurry to decrease or eliminate medications. Get the diet working first. Get the seizures under better control first. When the family and child are on a stable routine, one medicine at a time can be gradually reduced and, if there is no recurrence of seizures, eliminated. If medication is reduced in this systematic, gradual fashion and the child does have a few seizures, it becomes easy to figure out the reason. The key to weaning children off their anticonvulsant medications during the fine-tuning period is to separate the effects of decreasing doses of medications from other factors in the diet. In other words, don't reduce medications at the same time as adjusting the food. Also, if a child has breakthrough seizures while the medicine is being reduced, don't assume that the seizures are a result of the tapering off. Look for all the possible factors and try to determine whether the reduction in medication is the cause.

CARNITINE

There is a lot out there on the Internet about carnitine. In general, most people make enough carnitine to burn long chain fatty acids and do not need extra. However, we do check free carnitine levels at clinic visits, as do most ketogenic diet centers today. If the levels are <15, and especially if a child is sleepy or sluggish, extra carnitine (330mg capsules [or 3cc of the 1000mg/10cc solution], given three times a day) can be helpful. There is no proof that giving carnitine will also help reduce seizures. However, we all have a few cases where the parents say that it helped (although some may get worse). We will sometimes try a 1-month trial of carnitine for a child who had control on the diet but lost it over time. If it doesn't help, then we'll stop the carnitine.

FINE-TUNING THE MODIFIED ATKINS DIET

The modified Atkins is a lower ratio ketogenic diet that induces ketosis with less restrictiveness. Carbohydrates are reduced to 10 grams per day (20 grams per day for adults) and fats are encouraged. For more details see Section IV. Fine tuning details for this diet are provided in Chapter 19.

THE DECISION TREE

The first thing to look for when breakthrough seizures occur is whether the child has had an opportunity to eat something that is not on the diet. Someone may have given the child food or the child may have helped herself. One child was found to be sneaking sugared toothpaste in an upstairs bathroom. Another was slipping out of bed at night and raiding the refrigerator. Another girl had a seizure on Sunday, and her mother found to her dismay that a well-meaning grown-up at church had given her a lollipop.

Another possible cause of breakthrough activity on the diet is a calorie level that is set too high. If the body takes in more calories than are needed for maintenance, it will store those extra calories as fat. The body needs to burn all calories taken in to produce adequate ketosis and seizure control. Remember, the diet is simulating starvation, and you can't store calories when starving. As few as 100 calories too many per day can upset ketosis. In smaller infants, even 25 calories per day may be critical.

The level of urinary ketosis may vary with the time of day. It is usually lower in the morning and higher later in the day. This natural variation in the level of ketones as measured in the urine does not necessarily indicate a problem if it is not accompanied by seizures.

We will at times test the system in a child with low ketones by fasting the child for 24 hours. If the ketones rise after this fast, then we will decrease calories. With the exception of weight gain correlated to growth in height, weight gain on the diet is an indication that calorie levels are set too high. At an excess of 100 calories per day, it takes an entire month before any weight gain is seen. Therefore, some caloric adjustments can be made based on low ketone levels.

Sometimes better control may be achieved by using a 4.5:1 ratio for a period of time. The higher the diet ratio, the more restricted food options get, so the implications of raising the diet ratio should be seriously considered before it is prescribed.

> THE MOST COMMON cause of breakthrough seizures in a child who is getting the proper food and liquid levels is illness or fever.

An isolated seizure during illness requires no action on the part of the parents. Repeated breakthrough seizures can be the presenting sign of kidney stones, urinary tract infection, gastroenteritis, or other childhood infections. See Chapter 15 for greater detail on managing acute illness during the diet.

The ketogenic diet decision tree in Figure 12.1 can be used as a guide to investigating breakthrough seizures.

The Ketogenic Diet Decision Tree—for when a child with previous control begins having seizures.

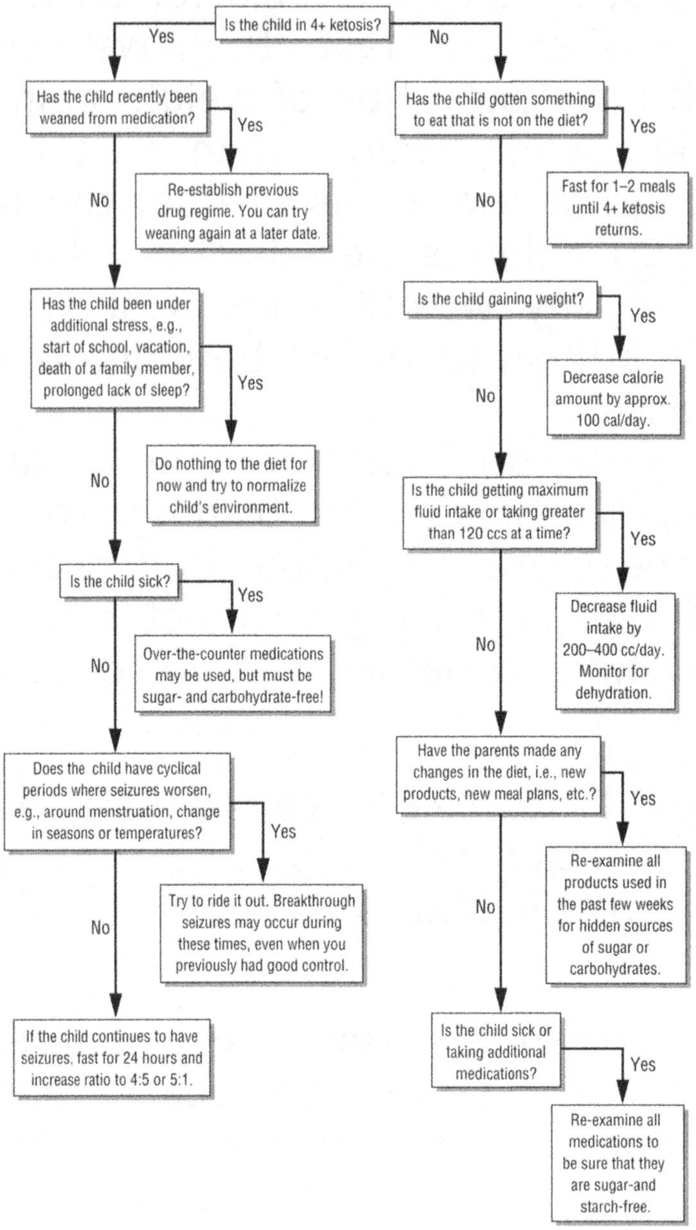

FIGURE 12.1

TOP TRICKS MONTHS AFTER STARTING THE DIET

Sadly, we also see children who come back after initially good seizure control and find that without any obvious diet-related problems (or illness), the seizures have returned. This is obviously disappointing and this "honeymoon" situation is frustrating for neurologists and dietitians as well. It is probably the number one reason we see children for consults from other ketogenic diet centers. Sometimes children just honeymoon to the diet as they had in the past to medications. However, there are some tricks we use, one at a time, to see if we can regain some control. Some have been mentioned earlier in this chapter already. They are listed in Table 12.2.

TABLE 12.2. Tricks to Regain Lost Seizure Control

- Lower (or sometimes raise) calories by 100 calories/day.
- Add carnitine (usually 330mg 3 times a day).
- Check serum anticonvulsant levels and increase them. Sometimes as children get bigger their levels will drift downward.
- Reduce anticonvulsants! Although this seems counterintuitive in children who are having more

seizures, sometimes it works. We have seen improvement, specifically in those on valproate and clonazepam, by reducing them.

• Fast occasionally for 12 hours (assuming the child has done this during the ketogenic diet admission before).

• Add MCT oil. In a way, this is a different diet (see Chapter 20) and might help.

• Increase temporarily to 4.5:1 (if at 4:1) or more permanently to 4:1. Realize, however, that studies to date show ratio changes months after starting the diet are not usually helpful.

• Lower the ratio! One of our previous dietitians Jane McGrogran, RD, taught us this trick. Again, it may seem counterintuitive, but some children do better at lower ratios with less ketosis.

• Spread out foods over the day. Sometimes ketones can dip if meals are too far apart.

THE LIMITS OF FINE-TUNING

In recent studies slightly more than half of children with difficult-to-control seizures find the ketogenic diet to be of sufficient benefit that they remain on the diet for more than 1 year. Not all of these are seizure free! A reasonable aim for parents as their child starts on the ketogenic diet is to achieve as much seizure control as possible with as few medications as possible.

Improvements in behavior, mood, mental alertness, and a general sense of well-being are additional benefits that the diet often brings. If parents set a goal of total seizure control, they may be setting themselves up for disappointment. Total control may not be possible.

After trying the diet for the initial 3-month period, and after working with the ketoteam to figure out if greater control can be achieved by adjusting food or medications, parents of children who have not responded to the diet or who have improved only moderately have to make a decision. These parents must weigh the benefits of the diet for their child against its burdens. Then they have to decide whether it is worthwhile for them to continue the diet.

CHAPTER THIRTEEN

Parent Support Groups and the Internet

Why this new chapter? Well, we found that most families found out in the past few years about the ketogenic diets, not from their neurologists, but from the Internet. There is a lot of good information out there from reputable sites that deal with epilepsy. The ketogenic diet parent support groups out there are growing in popularity, and their Web sites are usually the best places to get information and advice.

However, there's just as much misinformation. Some Web sites may have good intentions but share information that might have been true for one child on the ketogenic diet, but is not true for most others based on medical literature. Web rings and chat rooms have a habit of sharing bad stories at an equal rate to successes. Unfortunately, there are also people out there willing to give miracle cures to desperate parents at a high price, with little medical backing and no perceived responsibility for the risk. Be careful.

In general, the Internet *is* your friend. We advise our families to surf with caution, though, and *never* make any changes to the diet without checking with your ketoteam first. All neurologists and dietitians are busy, and the rapid replies many parents get from chat rooms and blogs can seem better. However, always discuss any advice you get with your neurologist and dietitian. They might surprise you and say, "That's a good idea!" They might also tell you that they've heard that advice before from other keto families and it led to disaster.

PARENT SUPPORT GROUPS

The Charlie Foundation

(www.charliefoundation.org)

FIGURE 13.1 Courtesy of the Charlie Foundation.

The Charlie Foundation was formed in 1994 at the time of the first edition of this book and was the first ketogenic diet support group. Created by Jim Abrahams, a movie producer from California, his son Charlie was treated at Johns Hopkins and became seizure-free rapidly (see the foreword to this book!).

His father was understandably upset at not being told about the ketogenic diet and then later being discouraged from using it. He created the movie *First Do No Harm* with Meryl Streep and helped support a 1996 Dateline NBC special. They also have supported research, such as a multicenter prospective study in 1998 (the first ever). The scientific advisory board of the Charlie Foundation meets annually at the annual American Epilepsy Society meeting in December and discusses how to continue to move the diets forward. These meetings have led to review articles and the 2009 expert consensus statement (see Chapter 11). The Charlie Foundation has also sponsored training sessions for many years for dietitians and neurologists and has been one of the major sponsors of the 2008 and 2010 international ketogenic diet conferences in Phoenix and Edinburgh, respectively. Beth Zupec-Kania has trained many international ketogenic diet center staff and runs KetoCalculator, used by many families on the ketogenic diet.

Matthew's Friends

FIGURE 13.2 Courtesy of Matthew's Friends.

(www.matthewsfriends.org)

Matthew's Friends was created in 2005 by Emma Williams and is the ketogenic diet support group for the entire United Kingdom. They also have branches in Holland and South Africa. Emma Williams formed Matthew's Friends along with many volunteers in response to her son Matthew, who had a similar experience as Charlie Abrahams. Matthew did well on the diet, and his mother created this support group to get the diet to more children not offered it previously. Similarly to the Charlie Foundation, they have sponsored many training sessions and the international ketogenic diet conferences. In addition, Emma has held parent days for both parents of children on the diet as well as those considering it—one in 2007 in London and 2010 in Edinburgh. Her Web site is full of useful information and updated frequently. They also have a scientific advisory board titled "KetoPAG."

The Carson Harris Foundation

(www.carsonharrisfoundation.org)

FIGURE 13.3 Courtesy of The Carson Harris Foundation.

This parent support group was created in Baltimore in 2007 by two parents, Gerry and Michael Harris, in response to the successful treatment of their infant daughter Carson at our center. Carson had infantile spasms and was offered the ketogenic diet as an initial treatment in addition to steroids and vigabatrin. The diet worked within days, and Carson was kept on the diet for 6 months total. She is now 5 years old and completely normal. The Harris family created the Foundation and ran a highly successful fundraiser (Carson's FeelGood Fest, with Adam Duritz of the Counting Crows) to fund research related to the ketogenic diet. Gerry Harris also now runs our Johns Hopkins parent support group and, along with about 20 other families, will chat with families during their ketogenic diet admission week. Their message of encouraging neurologists to offer the diet much earlier in the course of epilepsy is at the heart of their Foundation.

Epilepsy Cure Initiative

(www.epilepsycureinitiative.ca)

Epilepsy cure initiative

FIGURE 13.4 Logo is courtesy of ECI.

This support group is based in Toronto, Canada, and run by Margaret Maye (a successful and incredibly talented opera soprano!) and her husband, Gary Neumann. Their son, now an adult with epilepsy, was treated by the family with the ketogenic diet mostly on their own using computer programs with some success. They are committed to promoting the use of dietary treatments in Canada and have sponsored and organized ketogenic diet conferences for parents and neurologists.

Japan

(http://www2.ocn.ne.jp/~ketodiet/)

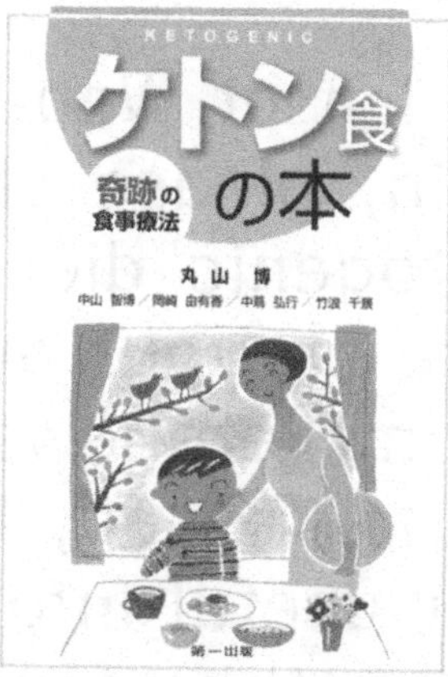

FIGURE 13.5 Courtesy of Hiroshi Maruyama.

Mr. Nakasuta, the father of a child with epilepsy who became seizure-free on the ketogenic diet, has created this group to increase awareness in Japan. Unfortunately, his son died several years ago due to an accident (not related to the diet). He has created a stunning recipe book in Japanese and is trying to increase awareness of the diet in Japan, especially to show that it can be adapted successfully to Asian lifestyles and food preferences.

Israel

(www.oliversmagicdiet.com)

Talia and Eli Berger have set up a parent support group in 2010 in Israel. Their son Oliver has Doose syndrome and has done extremely well on the ketogenic diet. Their goal is to increase awareness and dietitian training in Israel. The Web site, www.oliversmagicdiet.com, can be translated on Google.com from Hebrew.

Internet sites

This is a partial list of Web sites that we have found helpful. Again, please check anything you read with your ketogenic diet team first before following any advice on your own.

www.epilepsy.com/ketonews

A site run by Eric Kossoff, MD, on epilepsy.co m (which has other useful information on epilepsy). Includes a bimonthly newsletter (archived), recipes, lists of ketogenic diet centers worldwide and links.

www.hopkinsneuro.org

Johns Hopkins Pediatric Neurology Web site, with information on the ketogenic diet, Atkins diet, the adult epilepsy diet center

www.ketocalculator.com: KetoCalculator program

www.facebook.com (enter the group for Friends of Hopkins Ketogenic Diet Group)

www.charliefoundation.org: The Charlie Foundation for Epilepsy

www.matthewsfriends.org: Matthew's Friends

www.carsonharrisfoundation.org: The Carson Harris Foundation

www.atkins.com: Atkins Nutritionals Web site, with good tips and recipes

http://health.groups.yahoo.com/group/ketogenic/ :Yahoo.com site

www.myketocal.com

Information on KetoCal™, a ketogenic diet formula supplement

www.ketovolve.com

www.ketobake.com

www.epilepsyfoundation.org

Information about from the Epilepsy Foundation

modifiedmom.wordpress.com: created by a mother of a child on the modified Atkins diet

www.aesnet.org

American Epilepsy Society Web site

www.ilae.org

International League Against Epilepsy Web site

www.atkinsforseizures.com

A useful Web site created by the family of a child in our first pediatric Atkins study

www.specialcheese.com/bakedch.htm

Just the Cheese™ snacks

www.dukesmayo.com

High fat mayonnaise, very useful

www.bickfordflavors.com

No-carbohydrate flavorings

www.tomsofmaine.com

No-carbohydrate toothpaste

www.netrition.com

Useful for buying products, including MCT oil

www.carbsense.com

Makers of low-carb products with plenty of fiber; well-liked.

www.calorieking.com

Information on *The 2011 Doctor's Pocket Calorie, Fat & Carb Counter,* a helpful resource for modified Atkins patients.

CHAPTER FOURTEEN

Side Effects of the Ketogenic Diet

All therapies, both anticonvulsant medications and dietary manipulation, have either known or potential side effects. A great deal more has been learned the past few years, and will continue to be learned in the future, about what the unintended consequences of initiating and maintaining the ketogenic diet may turn out to be. Now in 2011, we are at the point of preventing side effects before they happen rather than treating them when they occur. The potential pitfalls and problems fall into four broad categories: pre-diet evaluation, issues during the initiation of the diet, short-term side effects while on the diet, and the long-term risks.

BEFORE EVEN STARTING

It is important to prevent side effects before they occur. One of the physicians on our ketoteam tries to schedule a face-to-face outpatient clinic visit with the candidate child and his parents/caregivers in almost every case. Nothing can substitute for the opportunity to personally interview parents, ask additional questions about the history that may not be available from the child's medical records, and examine the child.

There are exceptions, of course, especially when geographic issues are hard to overcome or the wait for a clinic appointment is much longer than the wait to start the diet. In those cases, we rely heavily on receiving "primary source" records, such as hospital discharge summaries, EEG and MRI data, and laboratory reports.

There are a few screening tests that must be documented. Most critical is to confirm that each child is not at significant risk for certain known metabolic conditions. This can be understood by performing studies such as lactate, pyruvate, and ammonia levels; plasma amino acids; and urine organic acids, if they are not already documented as normal. In many cases, a spinal fluid analysis will be obtained.

A careful history regarding food allergies should be completed. Because the diet for the most part consists of "normal" foods, the likelihood of problems in this area is low but must be screened for. It is possible for a skilled dietitian to design a diet even for children who have food allergies, and we have done so successfully many times.

Simply stated, the ketoteam and the parents/caregivers of the child who are considering dietary therapy must communicate clearly and come to an agreement that the "cost/benefit" analysis is favorable enough to proceed.

PROBLEMS DURING THE START OF THE DIET

Minor problems often arise during diet induction. That is why we still have all our patients in the hospital for this process over a 4-day admission. It should be noted that there are some centers that do start the diet as an outpatient procedure. We believe this can be done in very select families and with *very* careful monitoring (including daily visits to the outpatient clinic during the initiation period). In general, we advocate this primarily in situations where the risk of the child getting sick from another child in the hospital for something different is too high. We have also occasionally started the diet in children with well-established home nursing care where transport is problematic (e.g., children on ventilators or receiving many medications), but even in these situations there is constant daily contact.

There is controversy regarding the need to have children fast prior to starting to consume the diet. Over time, we have modified our protocol from a pre-diet 48 hour fast to only 24 hours. Exceptions are made for very young infants or children who are medically less stable, who do not fast at all. Fasting starts the night before admission so that it is more than half over by the time the child is on the hospital floor. Fasting clearly accelerates the onset of ketosis, and if carefully monitored in the hospital setting, does not put the child at significant risk. But studies show that there is no difference in long-term outcomes using fasting versus nonfasting protocols.

Hypoglycemia and acidosis

Fasting may lead to hypoglycemia. Blood sugars are monitored about every 6–8 hours during the first few days of the diet by dextrostix. We know that levels of 40–50mg/dl are not uncommon during diet induction and virtually never require a medical response. When blood sugar falls below 30mg/dl, the test is repeated in 1 hour. If the child becomes symptomatic—too sleepy or sweaty—30ml of orange juice may be given and repeated in 30 minutes if necessary. We avoid doing studies that require any type of sedation during this time to avoid possible confusion with hypoglycemia.

Acidosis can occur as well when the diet is started, and sometimes does persist. This can manifest as vomiting or sleepiness. We expect a child's bicarbonate level to fall when he or she becomes ketotic; this is typical when an acidosis condition is created in the body. If the bicarb level falls below 10mEq/L or pH falls below 7.2, then vomiting often occurs. We don't always check for this (requires a blood draw to the lab), but we presume it is happening based on clinical signs and will give extra fluids, sometimes including bicarbonate.

Dehydration

At the onset of ketosis after the fast, many children do not drink fluids at their usual rate. Therefore, we encourage "pushing" oral fluids that are carbohydrate free (water or diluted diet soda or ginger ale) during the fast and the entire hospitalization. We no longer measure and restrict fluid intake; there is no evidence for any benefit, and there is a slightly increased risk of dehydration. It is rare for a child to become so dehydrated that he requires a bolus of fluid to be given either intravenously (IV) or by nasogastric (NG) tube, but we do that on occasion if the vomiting is very severe.

Vomiting

After fasting for 24 hours, or even without it, the initial food intake, usually given as a "keto shake" or KetoCal®, may cause nausea and vomiting. This does not usually persist long and can be overcome by having the child take small sips of the shake over a relatively long period of time at the initial meal, as opposed to drinking it rapidly. We find that using the keto shake seems to be well-tolerated and less nauseating than if you went to straight ketogenic diet solid foods immediately. In some situations we will give Reglan®, Zofran®, or IV fluids. Children with reflux before the diet can have this more often on the diet, too, so be ready.

Refusal to eat

We introduce the total calorie load over 3 days, at a rate of 33% per day divided into three feedings. Thus, the first day, the allotment is one-third of calories, the next day two-thirds, and the last day 100%. Even though most of the children are very hungry after the fast, some respond to being ketotic by lacking a feeling of hunger. Some of them refuse to eat and need a lot of encouragement. It may require that the keto shake be sipped slowly over several hours, or frozen into "ice cream," or microwaved into "scrambled eggs," and eaten slowly. For other children, we'll advance the diet to solid foods a bit more quickly—going straight to regular foods rather than the keto shake a day or two early. However, the downside to this is that vomiting may occur.

SHORT-TERM SIDE EFFECTS WHILE ON THE DIET

Changes in weight

We now know that achieving a child's "ideal" body weight is no longer a crucial factor in the long-term success or failure of the diet. Optimal ketosis and seizure control are not usually weight dependent, and so you do not need to check weight frequently. However, if control is poor, or if control suddenly changes without a clear reason, knowing the child's weight may be a factor in the decision-making process for making diet changes.

In some children, a slight weight loss may be healthy and intentional.

Illness and infections

All children suffer intermittent illnesses, and there is no clear evidence to suggest that children on the ketogenic diet are more susceptible to infections than others. Should a child have an illness that requires IV fluids, parents need to make physicians and emergency room personnel aware that their child is on the ketogenic diet and that in almost every case, the IV fluids used should be completely sugar-(dextrose) and carbohydrate-free. The exception would be if a child is so dehydrated and acidotic that he or she has a hypolygemic seizure, at which time, of course, the child must be given glucose by IV. A general rule is that whenever the safety of a child is a serious issue, and medical treatment requires action that will diminish or end ketosis, that takes precedence over maintaining the diet. Remember, after a crisis is over, ketosis can always be reestablished, and the benefits of the diet reestablished.

Vitamin and mineral deficiency

The ketogenic diet is deficient in vitamins and perhaps in minerals as well. Severe examples are beri beri and optic neuritis due to lack of thiamine. Major minerals such as calcium and trace elements such as selenium are examples of those that are frequently deficient. All centers prescribe carbohydrate-free multivitamins and mineral supplements, which are readily available. Vitamin D, calcium, zinc, and selenium are important to make sure are included in the supplements (see Chapter 10).

Kidney stones

Overall, the risk of kidney stones while on the diet is increased and occurs in 1 in 20 children. The most common association is documented family history of kidney stones in the parents or siblings of the child on the diet. The medication type called carbonic anhydrase inhibitors (the common ones are Topamax® and Zonegran®) have a slightly increased risk of kidney stone formation but do not have to be discontinued when the ketogenic diet is started or maintained. Data are a bit controversial whether these medications increase the risk over the diet alone.

Kidney stones are generally calcium or uric acid stones, and the first indicator is usually the presence of traces of blood in the child's urine. Parents can check urine every other week for blood on the multistix test strip. Clinical symptoms of kidney stones may be as specific as frank blood in the urine, "gritty" urine, and/or lower back (so-called "flank") pain. Nonspecific symptoms include low-grade fever, abdominal pain, poor appetite, and an increase in number of seizures.

If kidney stones are suspected, carbohydrate-free fluids should initially be pushed hard to flush the urinary tract. If symptoms persist, the primary care physician needs to be consulted so that this possible complication can be differentiated from the much more common gastrointestinal virus or flu. The use of diagnostic abdominal ultrasound is recommended in cases where stones cannot be ruled out.

We now prescribe Polycitra K® or Bicitra® as soon as the diet is started for all children, regardless of known risk factors. These compounds raise the pH (technically called alkalinization) of the urine, which lowers the likelihood of stone formation by 7-fold (see Chapter 10). In most cases where stones are documented but small, they can be flushed out by increasing urine flow through increased carbohydrate-free oral intake or IV fluids. In rare cases, stones must be broken up by lithotripsy (using vibration) or even at times by surgery.

Constipation

This is one of the most common issues for children on the ketogenic diet, likely caused by a combination of reduced bulk in the diet and decreased fluid intake.

After the diet regimen is established, we expect children to have a bowel movement pattern similar to pre-diet. That should be a frequency of no less than once every other day and with normal stool consistency so there is no straining.

To help avoid digestive problems while the body gets used to the new diet, we recommend use of George's Aloe Vera® or Miralax® crystals (starting with one capful—about 17 grams daily) and expect parents to make adjustments over time to "keep things moving." Sometimes these products need to be used long term, and that is fine. Enemas can be used if necessary, but are rarely needed.

High cholesterol and other lipid abnormalities

We live in a society very concerned with total cholesterol levels, "good" and "bad cholesterol levels, and elevated triglycerides. Not surprisingly, when people learn that a child is being given a diet that is in excess of 80% fat, they are both surprised and concerned. Our study of lipid level changes on the ketogenic diet indicates that in about 30% of children there may be cholesterol and triglyceride levels "that exceed current recommendations for normal children," but in most cases this is a transient finding. As the body (primarily the liver) adjusts to the greatly increased load of fat it must digest when the ketogenic diet is started, the levels begin to stabilize and then return very close to pre-diet levels after 6–12 months. In cases where children experience exceedingly high lipid levels, there may be a coincident genetic type of familial hyperlipemia that was exacerbated by the high fat diet.

A study shows that in children on the diet for longer than 6 years, most of them had cholesterol levels in the normal range. When the diet is discontinued, and the child returns to a diet with a presumed "normal" fat intake, lipids almost always return to normal. We do not have any evidence that there are long-term effects of a temporary increase in lipids as a child.

What if the cholesterol won't come down? Reducing the diet ratio, increasing the percentage of polyunsaturated fats, substituting medium chain triglycerides, and adding carnitine are the most common approaches we take. However, a study here showed that although 60% of children have at least a 20% reduction in cholesterol by making some (or all) of these changes, about 40% had their cholesterol decrease by at least 20% with just observation alone. In other words, it may be best to just repeat the labs after 1–2 months and leave the diet alone.

We have had virtually no child discontinue the diet exclusively for lipid abnormalities, and have never yet treated a child on the diet who has markedly elevated cholesterol with statin medication.

Carnitine deficiency

Many children on the diet for several months, especially if on valproate (Depakote®) at the same time, will have a decrease in their free carnitine. According to the international consensus statement, these children should be then treated with Carnitor®. At our center, we only do that if the levels are low *and* the child is symptomatic (e.g., fatigue, low energy, low ketosis). There is more information on carnitine in Chapter 10.

LONG-TERM SIDE EFFECTS

Studies of children on the diet for over 6 years have shown that seizure control and cholesterol are not adversely affected over time. However, the bad news is that bone fractures, kidney stones, and height disturbance *are* more of a problem long term. This doesn't mean the diet has to be stopped, but it does mean that ketoteams need to be very aware of this and try to prevent problems before they occur.

There are definitely exceptions. A man in his 20s with tuberous sclerosis who has been on the ketogenic diet for nearly his entire adult life identified himself and presented to our clinic several years ago. He had no history of appetite or growth issues, kidney stones, constipation, or evidence of acidotic episodes. His bone density (DEXA) scan and carotid ultrasound were normal for his age. He remains on the diet, seizure free to this day.

Bone metabolism

Very debilitated, nonambulatory children who are on the ketogenic diet have a high incidence of bone changes that can be documented on radiologic studies and DEXA scans. We also know that vitamin D levels decrease over time (after initially going up on the diet due to the added supplements). We supplement 400–800 International Units per day of vitamin D when levels are demonstrably low Until they can be normalized and maintained at a lower dose. We do not routinely obtain skeletal X-rays or DEXA scans on our patients in the short term, but if they are on the diet over 2–3 years it is worth considering.

Changes in height

We expect children to grow normally in height while on the diet, although younger children may have a slight initial drop off of their growth rate. Studies have shown that the problems with height may be related to ketosis itself, so could happen as well with the modified Atkins diet, not just the ketogenic diet. Most children grow fine, but if they don't, there is evidence that there is growth "catch up" when the diet is discontinued.

When we see our patients periodically in follow-up clinic, we of course measure and chart their weight and height. We want to see weight increase and linear height growth over time, in context of the child being able to have as much seizure control as possible, continue everyday activities, and all the while remaining in good health. If there is a problem, we will often lower the ratio to increase protein, even to the extent of the modified Atkins diet. Some children on the diet around the world have been started on growth hormone, with early reported good results (no studies yet).

Miscellaneous complications

Included in this category are bleeding disorders, increased bruising, and hepatitis, which are all liver-related problems; pancreatitis; iron deficiency anemia; prolonged QT intervals (heart); and alteration in immunoglobulin levels and function leading to possible increased occurrence of infections. Most of these problems are easily recognizable with regular clinical and laboratory monitoring and are correctable when diagnosed using the accepted treatments currently available.

Death

There are rare case reports of deaths occurring that may be attributable to the ketogenic diet. These are due to cardiomyopathy, selenium deficiency leading to cardiac arrhythmia, secondary to aspiration of fatty food contents (usually liquid formulas) causing lipoid pneumonia. One of our patients died due to recurrence of a cardiomyopathy of unknown cause, which had been identified well before the diet was started. Some children sadly may die as well of SUDEP (sudden unexpected death in epilepsy patients), which is more common in those with frequent, generalized-tonic-clonic seizures, especially receiving many anticonvulsants.

SUMMARY

The ketogenic diet was not originally intended for long-term use as an epilepsy treatment, but because it has successfully reduced seizure frequency and improved general quality of life for so many patients, including infants, children, and adults, its usage has frequently been extended for many consecutive years. It is not alternative or, therefore, free of side effects. Thus, when patients, caregivers, and the ketogenic diet team embark on the difficult course that this therapy requires, we have accumulated enough experience and real data to help guide us through many of the pitfalls and issues that will likely confront us. And as time goes on, we will learn more, and hopefully optimize treatment and minimize the complications discussed in this chapter.

CHAPTER FIFTEEN

Making it Work at Home and on the Road

BE CREATIVE, but follow the rules exactly. Follow the rules exactly, but be creative.

As long as you follow the rules exactly, but think creatively, you and your child can do just about anything you ever did before the diet started.

TIME SAVERS

At first, most families find that the diet is very time-consuming to plan and prepare. But it gets faster and easier as you become accustomed to using the gram scale and planning meals in advance. We have estimated that in the first weeks, shopping and meal preparation may add an extra hour or two of commitment each day. But after this initial period, once you have gotten used to weighing food, parents say that preparing the diet may add a half-hour per day at most.

The first time preparing meals takes forever. I was nervous weighing the foods and making sure that Danny would eat it, but the second time was easier. Once I learned the foods that Danny likes, I was able to prepare his foods much quicker in the kitchen.

Preparing and storing meals or parts of meals in advance can save much time. You can refrigerate many foods for a few days or freeze them for months. Following are some time-saving tips from parents who have experienced the diet:

- I cut up his favorite vegetables and keep them in plastic bags in the refrigerator for a few days. Then I can take them out and weigh a meal in no time.
- I usually make cream popsicles once a week and freeze them. He has one after every dinner.
- We measure a day or two of meals at a time and put them in containers. That way we only have to do the weighing about every other day. Also, we can either serve the meals at home or take them with us if we are eating out.
- We make sure to label each ingredient that we have weighed, like "25g of cream for the egg and bacon meal," this way we know exactly which meal it belongs to.
- Whenever someone is celebrating a birthday at school, I know what to make for him—I send him in with a fruit-topped ketogenic cheesecake so he can have something good to eat, too.
- I put a cream shake in a container and freeze it so he can eat it later as ice cream or let it thaw back down to a shake.

- I always keep some tuna or chicken salad and bags of cut-up vegetables stored in the refrigerator in case I can't be there to fix dinner myself. He also takes these stored meals to school.
- We prepare grams of butter in little clear plastic cups, this way we can grab the butter and add it to his school lunch.

Be certain to label each meal or each part of a meal (Monday breakfast, Wednesday supper) before putting it in the refrigerator or the freezer so you remember what goes together.

GOING TO SCHOOL AND OTHER SHORT TRIPS

Anything the family did before, they can still do on the diet—it will just take a little more planning. Every parent who has been through the diet has suggestions to offer:

- The key to making the diet "portable" is reusable storage containers.
- Cold food is easier to transport than hot food.
- It is easy to get food microwaved in a restaurant.
- It is usually easier to weigh and assemble a whole meal or several meals at home in advance than to weigh food on the road.

WITH BOTH OF US WORKING, and with all of the sports and church things for the other kids, finding time to make Brian's ketogenic meals was very hard. We finally found that if his mom and

I worked together on Saturday morning, we could make all the meals for the week, label them, and put them in the freezer. Then at night we only had to make the family's supper—his was all ready to microwave.

Eggnog is the traditional replacement meal, designed for all-purpose substitution in case of travel, sickness, or emergencies that make it difficult to prepare a meal. Eggnog is a complete meal-in-one (except for vitamin supplements), which is part of what makes it so convenient. Most children like the taste. Each sip is ketogenically balanced, so they don't have to drink all of it, or drink it all at once, to get its ketogenic effect. Also KetoCal® or KetoVolve® can always be used on the road to provide a "shake" or milk drink, if the grams of powder are weighed beforehand than all that's required is to mix it with water. Macadamia nuts, sometimes mixed with butter to achieve a higher ratio (they are naturally 3:1), can also be used as a meal-in-a-pinch or a travel meal or snack. A bag of chopped macadamia nuts and a diet soda can be a very socially acceptable snack for older children to eat around their friends, for instance, on a field trip or sleepover.

Neither eggnog or macadamia nuts has enough protein nor the nutritional value of regular meals with meats, fruits, and vegetables. These are meant for snacks and should be used infrequently in place of meals. Both eggnog and macadamia nuts, however, can be extremely useful in a pinch.

We carried a small cooler with an ice pack in it everywhere. In the morning, we fixed the whole day's meals before going out. It got so that even if we weren't going anywhere we would set up all the meals for the day and stick them in Tupperware containers in the refrigerator. If we were going on a long trip, we would take about 2 days' worth of food with us in the cooler and bring our scale. Also, we always carried extra ingredients that we knew might be hard to buy, like olives. Everyone has a microwave, even on airplanes. We could give a fancy restaurant a couple of Tupperware containers and instructions for how long to cook things, and they would bring the food out on their own plate. Everybody was really co-operative.

The following are some meal ideas for taking to school or on short outings. Each meal requires several reusable containers for storage.

- Tuna, chicken, or egg salad with mayonnaise

  Fresh vegetables (cucumber, carrot, cherry tomato, celery) Sugar-free Jell-O with whipped cream
- Celery or cucumber boats stuffed with tuna salad, cream cheese and butter, or peanut butter and butter

  Vanilla cream shake, whipped and frozen overnight
- Sandwich rolled in lettuce (chicken, cheese, turkey, or roast beef with mayonnaise)

Water-packed canned peaches

Chocolate milk (cream diluted with water and flavored with pure chocolate extract and saccharin)

- Cottage cheese with chopped fruit or vegetables and mayonnaise

Cream shake, whipped and frozen overnight

- Fruit-topped "cheesecake," frozen overnight: a one-dish meal
- Soups in a thermos of chicken or beef, cream, butter, and vegetables
- Mac & cheese (Miracle Noodles) cheddar cheese, butter, and cream
- Greek salad with feta cheese, olives, and olive oil

Foods frozen overnight and taken out in the morning soften to a pudding-like consistency by lunchtime. Foods to be taken to school or on short outings can be wrapped in foil or carried in a thermal pouch or cooler for extra insulation to help stay either warm or cold. Whipped cream can be stored for a few hours and still keep its body.

> *When we went to Disneyland we just took a big cooler with 3 whole days of meals in labeled containers. Once we let him get a hot dog from the stand (which we then weighed) so he could feel like he was having a special treat. I wouldn't say it was easy doing all that planning, but for us it wasn't too difficult.*

If you are going out to eat at a restaurant and you want your child to have a hot meal, call first to make sure the restaurant has a microwave that can be used for heating your food. If you are giving the child a cold meal, ask the restaurant to bring out an extra plate, which will make the food look nice and add to the feeling of family togetherness. Most restaurants are very familiar with allergies and special diets. Many of them have heard of the Atkins diet, so use that to your advantage if they don't know what the ketogenic diet is. Their goal is to make you feel comfortable while eating in their restaurant, so if you call the restaurant ahead of time or if you speak to the Maître d', usually they will be able to prepare a plain piece of chicken breast or scrambled egg, and then you weigh out the food at the table.

DIET DON'TS

One mother kept her child out of school for a year and hired an in-home teacher because she did not want him to be tempted by seeing other children eat. Another family stopped going out entirely—no more McDonald's, no more Sunday dinners at Grandma's—until the child himself finally begged them, explaining that he would enjoy the atmosphere and would not be too tempted by the food. Another mother fed her child earlier and in another room so he "wouldn't feel different" from his siblings. We believe it is better to aim for inclusiveness, for living as normally as possible given the diet's restrictions. In our experience most children are able to participate in making the diet as much as possible a part of a normal, enjoyable life.

MANAGEMENT OF ACUTE ILLNESS DURING THE DIET

It may be difficult for a child who is sick to maintain ketosis. Sick children often do not feel like eating. Their activity level changes, and they don't burn as many calories when they are ill. For these and other reasons many children on the diet experience a decrease in their urine ketone levels when sick. Seizure activity may increase at these times, or breakthrough seizures may occur even in children who have been well controlled on the diet. Parents should rest assured that ketosis will become reestablished as the illness resolves. But seizures during illness are not solely due to a decrease in ketosis. For reasons that are not understood, children who have seizures and have never been on the diet are often more likely to have a seizure during their illness. It may be necessary to break ketosis in order to treat an illness effectively. The most important thing is to get your child well again. The diet can be resumed once your child is well. The following are general guidelines for caring for a sick child on the ketogenic diet. More information on other side effects of the diet is provided in more detail in Chapter 14.

After about 3 months on the diet we noticed my son was sleepy, refusing to eat, and fussy.

He doesn't speak, so we couldn't ask what was wrong. His ketones were 80 and he didn't seem dehydrated. We thought maybe the ratio was too high or calories needed adjusting? After a few days, we contacted our keto doctor who didn't think it had anything to do with the diet and suggested seeing our pediatrician. Fortunately, she figured out that he had an infected tooth and gums!

As seen in this example, it is important to remember that your child is still a child and can get sick. Not all problems while your child is on the diet are due to the diet!

VOMITING OR DIARRHEA

- Give only sugar-free clear liquids. Do not worry about restricting fluids. Offer them as frequently as tolerated.
- If vomiting lasts for more than 24 hours, use unflavored Pedialyte® to maintain electrolytes. Use for up to 24 hours (but not longer).
- When vomiting stops, you can introduce a 1/3 quantity eggnog meal. Each sip has the proper ketogenic ratio, and it is not necessary for your child to finish the eggnog if he or she does not want to. Increase as tolerated until the child is eating the full diet quantity, then resume regular menus.
- If your child becomes dehydrated and IV fluids are required, make sure that they are sugar-free

(normal saline, no dextrose). Physicians and nurses in emergency rooms are not thinking about the effects that glucose in the IV might have on the diet and on the child's seizures. If blood glucose is below 40mg/dl, a single bolus of glucose (1 gram per kilogram of body weight) may be given.
- If your child is using MCT oil in the diet, discontinue it until the illness is resolved. Substitute 1 gram canola or corn oil for each gram of MCT oil. The MCT oil can be resumed when your child is well.

FEVER

- Give sugar-free fever-reducing medicine. Acetaminophen suppositories are an excellent fever reducer that won't interfere with the diet.
- Offer sugar-free liquids without restriction while your child has a fever.
- If an antibiotic is needed, make sure it is sugar-free and sorbitol-free. Speak with your pediatrician about using injectable antibiotics when possible, as a 7- to 10-day course of oral antibiotics may interfere with ketosis.

TOO MUCH KETOSIS

Sometimes a change in the diet or illness can cause children to get into too much ketosis. Some signs of too much ketosis are:
- Rapid, panting (Kussmaul) breathing
- Irritability

- Increased heart rate
- Facial flushing
- Unusual fatigue or lethargy
- Vomiting

If you suspect your child may be in too much ketosis, give 2 tablespoons of orange juice. If the symptoms persist 20 minutes after giving the juice, give a second dose of 2 tablespoons orange juice. If the second dose of juice does not improve your child's condition, call your pediatrician and the supervising physician of your child's ketogenic diet immediately.

If you cannot reach the doctors, take your child to the emergency room. The emergency room doctors will check how acidotic your child has become. Intravenous fluids may be needed or even a dose of IV glucose to break up the excessive ketosis. In the meantime, ask the emergency room to continue trying to contact your ketoteam.

BABYSITTER MEALS

In most households, the person who usually prepares the meals is occasionally unavailable—working late, sick, at a party, or otherwise engaged. Not to worry! With a little planning, someone else can easily put a meal together from your prepared ingredients. Many parents store measured ingredients or prepared food a couple of days ahead of time in the refrigerator even when they are planning to be present to prepare each meal. The habit of preparing meals in advance both saves time on a routine basis and makes it easier to cope with special situations. Just like with nonketogenic meals, it rarely hurts to have something ready in the freezer.

LONG TRIPS

Yes, the family can take vacations. Longer trips by necessity involve more planning than shorter ones. Many families who take long vacations choose to stay in places where they can cook, such as friends' condominiums or motels with kitchenettes, rather than in hotels. They sometimes take eggnog for the road instead of a solid meal. They take their scale and call ahead to make sure that places where they will be staying have heavy cream and a microwave available. With the scale, they can order grilled chicken, steamed vegetables, and mayonnaise and create a quick meal right at the restaurant.

Families take coolers full of prepared ingredients for the first couple of days of a trip, and perhaps staples such as artificial sweetener and mayonnaise. If they are staying in a hotel with no kitchen, they might take a camping stove to cook on. They take a lot of storage containers and the calcium and multivitamin supplements, too, of course—they never forget those.

Apart from the nuisance of planning, the diet should be no obstacle to family fun. There is no reason why a child should not live a rich, full, and healthy life while on the ketogenic diet. There is no reason to deprive yourself or the rest of the family.

> *He skied this year for the first time in ages. He skied like you wouldn't believe. He's swimming, he's playing ball. He's definitely had a happier life on the diet.*

BE CREATIVE

Being creative can mean compensating for a small quantity of cucumbers and carrots by slicing them in tall, thin strips and fanning them out to cover more plate space. Using smaller plates can also make the food seem like more. It can mean dressing up the cream as a toasted almond ice cream—whip into a mound, flavor with almond extract and sweetener, and sprinkle with a crushed almond. Let the child sprinkle on the nuts for fun.

There are lots of calorie-free ways to keep the food lively. Play with variables that add interest, not calories:

- Shapes (molds and cookie cutters can help here)
- Natural food colors or food coloring
- Herbs and spices (just a tiny pinch because these have carbohydrates)
- Pure flavoring extracts
- Pretending

Of course, many children do not care about variety and whimsy in their food. Some children are comforted by regularity. We have seen many families cook the same six meals over and over for 2 years, and the children were perfectly content.

We freeze his diet decaffeinated pop in miniature ice cube trays. They make refreshing little treats. He has a small amount as a goodie before bedtime. We give it to him in a wine glass to make it fancy and special. We also make popsicles out of his pop. If it's clear pop, we let him mix in food coloring drops, so he is not only involved but also learning. This adds lots of laughs when his teeth and lips turn green or blue or purple.

Peaches can be swapped for strawberries, broccoli for spinach. Combine fruits or vegetables for variety—peaches with a couple of raspberries on top, or asparagus with carrots. Switching the foods around helps add variety to the meals. If a child wants variety, there's plenty of room for creativity within the diet.

He has his special "pizza." It's just cheese and ground beef melted on a thin slice of tomato, cut into triangles the shape of pizza slices. But he loves it. It's pizza to him!

FOLLOW THE RULES EXACTLY

If the recipes and quantities as prescribed by a dietitian are followed exactly, the family will know the child was given the best possible chance to obtain the maximum benefits of the diet. Being very strict helps the ketoteam know where a child stands with the diet and minimizes any confounding factors. The effect of the ketogenic diet is directly related to the food that is eaten. This may seem obvious, but it is the factor that makes the diet work.

Especially when using commercial products, knowing the precise content of the food is essential. Buy the exact brand specified by the dietitian. The same product, such as bologna, made by different manufacturers may have very different proportions of protein, fat, and carbohydrates. The dietitian will have based diet calculations on the proportions of a given brand, so if a new brand is used, the calculations may have to be changed.

If a different brand needs to be introduced, the parents or dietitian must research the product carefully, even if it means calling the manufacturer to find out. There may be information in KetoCalculator about this (Chapter 9). Make sure that the new brand is properly calculated into the meal plans.

> *It would never have occurred to us to eat something that wasn't allowed on the diet. Even when we were allowed to, when the diet was ending, we had a hard time imagining eating food that hadn't been allowed before.*

Even when a commercial product is known and used regularly, formulations and commercial recipes can change. If breakthrough seizures develop, this should be one source of suspicion. At the risk of repeating ourselves, ingredients of commercially prepared foods, which are beyond your power to control, have to be watched very carefully. Be cautious in reading labels as well. By law, products that contain less than 1 gram of an ingredient per serving may be listed as 0, so a product that you thought had no carbohydrates may actually have up to 0.9 grams. If used on a regular basis, this can add up to a lot of excess carbohydrates.

With basic ingredients such as fresh meat, fruit, and vegetables, this is not much of a problem, although the exact content of even fresh produce does vary slightly from one source to another. If your child is having problems with the diet, always consider the food—both its quantity and its content—as the most likely culprit.

Are there commercial products in the diet? Has the source of cream or bacon changed? Is the cream still 36–40% fat? Different children have different amounts of tolerance for variations in food content. It is the little things that can mean the difference between success and failure of the diet. If your child is doing well on the diet, obviously you shouldn't worry. You should simply continue to be careful.

> *There was one time we wanted to try a new brand of sausage. We read the label very carefully and checked it with Mrs. Kelly and everything. But shortly after we started including it in her diet, our daughter began feeling shaky, what she described as "wobbly" inside. Dr. Freeman said it sounded like she might be trying to breakthrough with seizures. We're pretty sure it was because of that sausage; either the*

label was wrong or it referred to raw quantities and we were using cooked, or something. We went back to the old brand, and then she was fine.

GET THE WHOLE FAMILY INVOLVED

When you and your child are making the tremendous effort to stick to the diet in pursuit of a tremendous goal, you need everyone's cooperation and encouragement. You can weigh the food in advance, but if you are not there at dinnertime, someone else—an older sister or brother, a sitter, a grandmother—can put it in the microwave and serve the meal.

A child on the diet and all the child's sisters and brothers, relatives, friends, and teachers should understand that even tiny amounts of cheating can spoil the overall effect of the diet and that their friendship, support, and encouragement are crucial to its success. It helps if family members avoid eating carb-rich foods in large quantities around the child, especially if the child is just starting and adapting to the diet.

Sarah had been on the diet for 2 weeks when her sister Grace had a birthday party. We didn't want to exclude her, so we made a special ketogenic diet pizza for her and she ate it the same time as the other children. When the other children wanted to eat candy and cake, we just brought Sarah outside and did another activity. Later, she came back inside and joined in games when they were finished eating.

YOU CAN MAKE THE DIET work for you and your family! Being creative, careful, and planning meals in advance goes a long way!

CHAPTER SIXTEEN

Going Off the Diet

You are coming to the end of what may have been a long journey. We know this is tough for any family. For children who are seizure-free, there is anxiety and fear about seizures coming back. For children who are not improved with the diet, there is sometimes a sense of depression at this having been the "last resort" (which it is not!). For those in between (50–99% improved), it's a mix of all those emotions.

In prior editions of this book, this chapter was brief and there was little real research to guide our recommendations. That has changed. We can be more specific about the odds. Despite that, every decision is a difficult one and needs to be made as a team approach: parents, neurologists, and dietitians together. Make only one change at a time. Do not wean the diet and medications at the same time! You also do not need to add a medication if the diet is being weaned. We are also generally not in favor of weaning the diet before big life events, trips, school examinations, and so forth. Plan ahead—in most situations, weaning the diet is not an emergency. Also make sure to have your neurologists' phone number or email readily available in case the wean does lead to worse seizures.

WHEN TO STOP THE DIET?

This question is truly up to the parents of the individual child. We will rarely "give up" on the diet in less than a month unless seizures are worsening or the child is having serious metabolic problems we can't fix. The data would suggest the diet will start to work within 4–6 weeks in most children (if it *is* going to work). However, we usually tell parents to give it at least 3 months just in case their child is a "late bloomer."

If it does work, there is no set time in which the diet must be stopped either. Even in super successful cases, most centers will start seriously considering the risks of the diet compared to benefits after 2 years. In many children, we suspect the diet has "done its job" and without it seizures will be no different than with it. The only way to find out ultimately is to wean the diet! For some children, the suspicion will be correct: Seizures will be no different. For some, it will not be: Seizures will get worse. Of course, it is important to be in close contact during the diet wean and have a plan already in mind for what to do if the seizures do worsen.

Some children who have responded exceptionally well to the diet start to come off it before the 2-year mark is reached. This decision is often suggested by the parents and agreed to in consultation with the physicians. We have done this in cases of Doose syndrome and infantile spasms especially, sometimes even after 6–12 months. For children with infantile spasms we treat before medications, if the diet works, we stop after 6 months.

Can the diet be continued longer than 2 years? Yes! The child who has had a good, but incomplete response to the diet and for whom the diet is not a burden may continue the diet on a visit-by-visit basis. We have had children who have remained on the diet as long as 26 years. A lot depends on side effects, too. But many families find the diet is easy and part of their routine ... and their child needs to eat anyway! The parents are really the primary decision makers at our center in determining when to stop the diet.

> *Ben has been on the diet for 9 years now. He is severely retarded and fed by gastrostomy. His cholesterol is 116. He has had no seizures in more than 8 years. Taper the diet? Why would we do that? The diet is no trouble for us and makes no difference to Ben.*

THE DOWN-SIDE OF LONG-TERM DIET USE

The long-term consequences of remaining on the ketogenic diet for many years have been recently studied, and although most children do very well, there can be problems. We recently studied about 30 children who had been continually on the ketogenic diet for 6–11 years. The risk of kidney stones and fractures is about 1 in 4 with this long-term use, so this needs to be closely watched, but no child had very significantly elevated cholesterol levels (above 400mg/dl). Studies have shown that lipids and triglycerides are elevated during the diet to levels that would normally be considered to increase the threat of stroke or heart disease after a lifetime of exposure. Bone fractures do occur more often in children on the diet for over 6 years (1 in 5). The potential threat of stroke or heart disease after a limited exposure of 2 or even 10 years of a high-fat diet does not appear to occur. Any health threat would have to be evaluated in relation to alternative health risks posed by uncontrolled epilepsy, such as increased seizures or increased long-term intake of anticonvulsant medications, but it is important for the clinician and family to weigh out the pros and cons of remaining on the diet. It may be important to test and see what the diet is still doing 5 years down the road by coming off of the diet. Many parents are scared to take their child off of the diet, but it is not a treatment without risks, and it has to be discussed yearly at each clinic visit to decide whether or not remaining on the diet for many years is beneficial to that patient.

> *I had not seen or heard from jack in many years when his family called to ask if they could increase his calories. We asked them to come to the clinic. Jack was now a late teenager, with cerebral palsy and moderate retardation. He had been on the diet for 15 years. He had grown and*

was doing well but still had one or two seizures per year. We decided to taper him off the diet, and after 6 months, he successfully came off it. Seizures did not worsen despite him being on no anticonvulsant drugs at the time of the wean.

HOW DO I WEAN THE DIET?

Previous editions of this book and even the 2009 consensus statement suggested that weaning the diet over "several" months was "traditional," but there has never been proof that slow wean was best. It is usually tapered so slowly as there is concern that a quicker discontinuation would lead to dramatic worsening (e.g., some children who may cheat with carbs and have a seizure). However, we have all seen children stop the diet abruptly during a hospitalization or emergency and do fine. In some children we would taper the diet by lowering the ratio every few days. They also would often do perfectly fine.

In the summer of 2010 Ms. Lila Worden, a Johns Hopkins medical student, looked at our experience in how to discontinue the diet—the first time this has ever been done. Interestingly, how it was done was different depending upon who the Hopkins neurologist was! About a third of the time it was stopped in 1–7 days. Another third was stopped over 1–6 weeks. The other third was more traditional, and the diet weaned over several months. In general, as would seem obvious, the children weaned slower tended to be those who had done better (i.e., seizure free and fewer medications at the time of the wean). If the diet didn't work, parents were anxious to stop it—as soon as possible.

The big surprise was that it didn't matter how quickly the wean was done. For 1 in 10 children, seizures get worse (>25% increase in seizures), no matter the speed of the wean. Details from this study are in Table 16.1.

These results have changed how we wean the diet—we are much quicker in weaning the diet than we used to be. Tapering the diet over months no longer seems necessary—we now typically will reduce the ratio every 1–2 weeks. If a child is in the hospital in a safe setting, generally for an emergency problem, we may discontinue the diet abruptly, too.

Our current recommended wean (for most children on a 4:1 ratio) is presented in the following list:

Weeks 1–2:	Reduce to 3:1
Weeks 3–4:	Reduce to 2:1
Weeks 5–6:	Reduce to 1:1 (modified Atkins)
Weeks 7–8*:	1:1 ratio, but unlimited calories
Weeks 9–10*:	Give high carbohydrate foods back, one meal at a time

*Check ketones daily during this weaning process. Remain on multivitamin, calcium, and oral citrate supplements during the wean. Keep in close contact with your ketogenic diet team! Can make these changes weekly, if desired.

Meals with lower ketogenic ratios are increasingly similar to regular meals. A 1:1 ratio will seem almost like a normal diet compared with the 4:1. There will be room for a lot more meat and vegetables and even the possibility of some carbohydrates.

Once a child has been weaned down to a 1:1 ratio and has been on that ratio for 1–2 weeks, we recommend that calories can be given ad lib (as much as desired). Then after 1–2 weeks, formerly forbidden foods can be gradually introduced into the diet. In general, as this happens and gradually introduced high carbohydrate foods have reached a point where the child is no longer in ketosis, and if seizures are stable (or still gone)—you're home free!

TABLE 16.1 Number Who Worsened by Discontinuation Rate

Outcome	Immediate (1–7 days)	Quick (1–6 weeks)	Slow (>6 weeks)
Overall	11%	11%	19%
<50% seizure reduction	3%	9%	9%
50–99%	26%	22%	36%
Seizure free	25%	9%	10%

If seizures worsen with the last few steps, we generally will go back to a 1:1 ratio. This is close to the modified Atkins diet (Chapter 18). We have many children in whom this happened, and they stayed on the modified Atkins diet for an additional several months to years. They generally found it easier than the ketogenic diet and were willing to keep carbohydrates reduced.

WILL MY CHILD GET WORSE DURING THE WEAN?

Back in 2007, we looked at this question for children who were seizure-free and stopped the diet. Thirteen of 66 (20%) had seizures return, sometimes years later. The seizures were most likely to come back in those who had (1) an abnormal EEG around the time of the wean, (2) an abnormal MRI for any reason (e.g., stroke or brain malformation), or (3) tuberous sclerosis complex. That doesn't mean we don't try to wean the diet in these seizure-free children—but we do it carefully. This year, Ms. Worden looked to see if any factors led to seizures worsening in *all* keto children (not just those seizure free). The only factor that seemed important was having a 50–99% seizure reduction. Children who were either seizure free or <50% improved rarely got worse. When she looked at those children specifically with 50–99% improvement, the only factor that seemed more likely to lead to seizures getting worse was being on more anticonvulsant drugs (1.4 vs. 0.8).

In other words, if your child is still having seizures on the diet after a few years but is definitely better, he/she is at a bit higher risk to have seizures worsen. There is a higher risk if they are on more seizure medications. You can try to wean the diet, just do it carefully!

TOWARD THE END we started letting him smell things. The other kids would give him a sniff of what they were eating, and he would say, "I can have that when I'm off the diet, right?"

SHE WAS A JUNIOR BRIDESMAID at a wedding the day she went off the diet. That was when she was 12. We had checked with Mrs. Kelly and agreed to let her eat cake at the reception. All of us were very apprehensive. There had been a lot of anxiety each time we cut the ratio, but she kept doing well, so sweets were the last test. Nobody else at the reception really knew what we were going through—it was a private thing among us and our very close friends. When she ate the cake and had no problems, it was thrilling for us. After that we were probably cautious for another week or two. Now she won't look at whipped cream, but she eats just like a typical teenager—pizza and candy and all the typical teenage food.

WE HAD BEEN DOWN TO A 1:1 RATIO for a few months when one day the doctor said, "Why don't you take him out for an ice cream sundae—you're off the diet!" Well, I couldn't quite do that but we did take him for a steak and potato dinner. Then about an hour later I got him a little dish of mint chocolate chip ice cream. It was very dramatic for me to see him eat a real meal. And for him, too—his little eyes were watering. It was a tear-jerking experience. We had finally made it! He used to be an extremely picky eater, but now he just really enjoys eating.

AFTER HE HAD DONE PERFECTLY for a year and a half on the 4:1 diet, we had done 6 months on the 3:1, and then a couple of months on the 2:1, when his sixth birthday was coming up. We asked him what he wanted, and he said pizza. Well, you're nervous as can be, but he was doing so well that we decided to stop the diet on his birthday, before the full 6 months of the 2:1 were up. We invited all the neighborhood kids in, and I put candles in the pizza. After he took the first bite, he looked up at me and said, "Dad, this is the best birthday present I've ever had."

ANXIETY AND RELIEF

It is natural for a parent to feel anxious when a child is going off the diet. After all that time spent planning and measuring food to an accuracy of a gram, it's hard to kick the habit! All we can tell nervous parents is that ending the diet is to their child's advantage once the child is seizure free for 2 years. The ketogenic diet therapy's goal is to treat a problem—seizures. Once the problem is gone, the therapy should also end.

GOING OFF THE DIET WAS VERY LIBERATING. At last we could go places without planning and thinking about every meal. We could spend a day at the mall. She could go to parties and eat what the other kids were having. It was great. We still see our neurologist, but it's in regular epilepsy clinic every few months. We ran into our dietitian at the mall several years later and gave her a big hug!

We know this is a tough moment for you. The diet is not like anticonvulsants—it requires lots of time and energy from parents and children. It also requires lots of work by the neurologists and dietitians who use it. We also find it hard to take our patients off the diet, and yes, we're nervous too! Our final advice is this: (1) one change at a time, (2) keep in close contact with your ketoteam, and (3) have a plan just in case the seizures get worse. Good luck!

SECTION IV

Modified Ketogenic Diets

CHAPTER SEVENTEEN

When and Why Should I Use Alternative Diets?

What is an alternative diet anyway? When we talk about alternative diets, we are referring to the modified Atkins diet (MAD) and low-glycemic index treatments (LGIT). These diets were invented in the early 2000s and were briefly touched upon in the 4th edition of this book. They are now much more widely used and deserve a section to themselves. Note: The MCT diet is a way to get fat in a slightly different way than the classical ketogenic diet and is not considered alternative per se (covered in Chapter 20).

The key benefit to these diets, and primary difference, is to achieve seizure control but in a less restrictive way. Both diets are similar to each other and also similar to the ketogenic diet; both require medical supervision. We look at them as more tools in your toolbelt, rather than competition. Similarities include high fat, low carbohydrate, and usually slightly lower calories (because it's hard to eat that much fat independently). Both the MAD and LGIT do need commitment from a parent and family, as well as the child. They still will be eating different foods, and their lifestyle will change somewhat. Cookies, candy, and cupcakes are still pretty much forbidden.

Eggs, bacon, and cream are still encouraged (although a bit less so with the LGIT). Labs including cholesterol need to be checked before starting and every few months.

Jordan was a 4-year-old boy with seizures in a family of six living in an Amish community. The family ate in large groups and was very concerned that eating separately would make Jordan self-conscious. In addition, they were worried about the hospital admission for the diet and how their other children would be cared for during a hospitalization. They had also never slept in a hospital before. After a long discussion and talking to other families, they decided to try the modified Atkins diet first. If that wasn't helpful, they were given the option to switch to the traditional ketogenic diet. Jordan did great and had excellent seizure control; he never needed to switch after all.

These diets do have differences, primarily in regard to strictness. They allow more carbs and protein, and calories are not carefully monitored. Both are started in the clinic without a fast. Neither diet requires gram scales or weighing of foods, although portion sizes are important to know. We do not know for sure if side effects are fewer, but in our experience so far they seem to be a bit less, especially in terms of the child's growth and development of kidney stones.

HOW CAN I CHOOSE?

Every child and every family is different. There is no right or wrong answer to which diet your child (or you) should start. The best thing to do is read this book and information on the Internet about these diets and look at recipes. Talk to other families that have done it and ask them. Making a decision does not mean you are stuck with one diet; you can always switch between them if necessary (more on that later in the next chapter). Our current general decision tree is described in the next section.

DECISION ALGORITHM FOR DECIDING BETWEEN KETOGENIC AND MODIFIED ATKINS DIET AT JOHNS HOPKINS HOSPITAL

Jamie was a 3-year-old girl who was started on the low-glycemic index treatment by her local neurologist and dietitian. Although it led to 50% reduction in her seizures, her mom and dad never felt they had a good grasp on how to do it, and often worried they were "doing it wrong." After a year, they were admitted and started on the ketogenic diet. There was no change in her seizures, but her mom and dad found the ketogenic diet "easier" in some ways as they were given very specific meal plans by the dietitian, and there was less stress due to worry about making the wrong foods. After a year on the ketogenic diet, the family requested switching back to the low-glycemic index treatment to make it a bit easier on Jamie as she found the ketogenic diet tough. This time around, her mom and dad were "pros" and found it much easier.

There are some situations in which we do not generally recommend "alternative" diets, and tell families to go to the traditional ketogenic diet. One situation is children with gastrostomy tubes. There is no "Atkins" formula—ketogenic diet formulas (see Chapter 8) are easy to use and come in 3:1 or 4:1 ketogenic ratios. Therefore, there is no advantage to the modified Atkins diet for these children in being less restrictive. The formula could be made into a 1:1 or 2:1 ratio if necessary as well. A second situation is an infant. Besides the availability of ketogenic formulas, infants are a bit more "high risk," and we feel the careful calculations of calories and protein with the ketogenic diet may add a level of supervision that is needed for these patients. Similarly, any child with nutritional compromise or fragility may be better served with the close dietitian support of the ketogenic diet. Lastly, families in which there is an obvious need for the extra help and guidance of a dietitian in creating meal plans and recipes do better with the ketogenic diet. Although the alternative diets allow flexibility, we have some families that find it too "vague" or "uncertain" and prefer the unequivocal nature of the ketogenic diet.

The most important thing that we cannot emphasize enough is that no matter what diet you choose to start, you should do it with a neurologist and preferably dietitian available. All of us in the ketogenic diet community have seen disasters where children are started on an "alternative" diet thinking it's easy and simple, but are either given no support or misleading information. If you read something on the Internet that seems wrong, or your neurologist or dietitian seems confused about something related to the diet, pause and double check. There is nothing worse than a child doing poorly on a diet started by the parents and parents forever thinking that diets will not work. They are often upset years later when it is retried and much more successful.

CHAPTER EIGHTEEN

The History of the Modified Atkins Diet for Epilepsy (and Future Directions)

THE PIONEER PATIENTS

A 9-year-old boy was on the ketogenic diet since age 5 for his intractable absence type seizures. However, he had significant behavior problems, which the diet was helping, but it still became difficult to keep him on the diet. In August 2001, on her own, his mother switched him to the Atkins diet. His seizures remained under control with less episodes of cheating. Seizures worsened when his mother added carbohydrates, so our natural impulse was to put him back on the stricter ketogenic diet. After 2 more years of dealing with food battles, his mother switched him back for the second time to the Atkins diet, which he remains on still to some degree today, now 10 years in ketosis.

In March 2003, a young 7-year-old girl was 1 month away from her scheduled week-long admission for the ketogenic diet. Her seizures were occurring 70–80 times per day, and she had failed 8 anticonvulsants. In preparation for the ketogenic diet, we suggested a gradual reduction of high-carbohydrate items, such as bread, pizza, cake, and breakfast cereal in order to get the child used to the foods that would be given. Her mother asked for more information to help reduce carbohydrates, so we suggested buying *Dr. Atkins' New Diet Revolution* and reading about the induction phase. That was Friday; by Monday her seizures had totally stopped.

Needless to say, we were shocked. When we saw her in clinic later that week, her urine ketones were large. Our dietitian calculated she was receiving about 10 grams per day of carbohydrates, which we recommended she continue. We also started a multivitamin and calcium and began to check cholesterol periodically. After 1 month of seizure freedom, we cancelled her admission for the diet. She remained on the modified Atkins diet for about 4 years before seizures returned and she eventually stopped it to pursue epilepsy surgery (which did eventually lead to seizure freedom).

After these first two children, others were tried on a modified Atkins diet of 10 grams/day of carbohydrates. Details of these children and some adults can be found in the next chapter. Although the induction phase of the Atkins diet allows 20 grams/day of carbohydrates, our dietitian believed that the ketogenic diet generally allows 5–10 grams/day, and therefore 10 grams/day was a more appropriate starting point for children. She felt the Atkins diet was likely approximating a 1.5:1–2:1 ratio.

IS THE ATKINS DIET THE SAME AS THE KETOGENIC DIET?

Since the Atkins diet creation in the 1970s, families that were told to start the ketogenic diet often asked "Is this the Atkins diet?" Our typical answer was "Of course not!" Although we were quick to point out the many differences, there were just as many similarities.

The Atkins diet was created in the 1970s by the late Dr. Robert C. Atkins as a means to combat obesity. It has become very popular since the year 2000, as a result of several high-profile articles in the *New England Journal of Medicine,* the clear failure of the obesity epidemic to improve with the "accepted" low-fat diet, and the widespread availability of pre-packaged low carbohydrate snacks and meals in stores and restaurants. Similar to the ketogenic diet, it encourages fat intake and restricts carbohydrates. Foods on the Atkins diet are very similar to what is eaten on the ketogenic diet. Both diets can induce weight loss, although with the Atkins diet, it's the major goal compared to the ketogenic diet! For many years the medical community described both diets as voodoo medicine, unsafe, unlikely to work, and dangerous ... but has recently changed their minds.

TYPICAL 2 DAYS OF FOOD FOR A CHILD ON 10G/DAY MODIFIED ATKINS DIET

Day 1

Breakfast

Scrambled eggs
Bacon (2 strips)
36% heavy whipping cream diluted with water to make milk

Lunch

Bologna/ham, lettuce, Dijon mayonnaise "roll-ups"
Raspberries (1/2 cup)
Cucumber slices (1/2 cup)
Flavored, calorie-free, sparkling water

Snack

Just the Cheese™ (crunchy) snacks

Dinner

Hot dog
Spaghetti squash with butter and salt (1/4 cup)
Sugar-free flavored Jell-O™ topped with whipped heavy cream

Day 2

Breakfast

Sausage links
Low carbohydrate yogurt
Water

Lunch

Cheeseburger (no bun)
Cole slaw
Pickle
Heavy whipping cream, water, and unsweetened cocoa powder

Snack

5 macadamia nuts
Mozzarella cheese stick

Dinner

Sliced chicken, coated in egg and CarbSense™ baking mix then fried in olive oil

Steamed, mashed cauliflower with salt, butter, and pepper (mashed "potatoes")

1/2 cup of strawberries topped with heavy whipping cream

The big similarity between the two diets: *ketosis.* Throughout the book *Dr. Atkins' New Diet Revolution,* there are references to using urine ketone strips to monitor ketosis as a sign of burning fat and weight loss. In fact, in the "induction phase" of the Atkins diet, 20 grams/day of carbohydrates is advertised as leading to a ketotic state, but above that would not. The high levels of ketosis, although surprising to us, turned out to be no surprise to the Atkins Foundation. When contacted, they were extremely friendly and helpful with information.

IS THE MODIFIED ATKINS DIET DIFFERENT THAN THE KETOGENIC DIET?

Yes. There are many important differences between the modified Atkins diet and the ketogenic diet. They are listed in Table 18.1. It has less fat and more protein and carbohydrates, but still it's different than the standard diet. The modified Atkins diet does not restrict protein or calories and can be started without a fast or hospital admission. Certainly some centers do not fast or admit their children, but the modified Atkins diet can be started quickly in the clinic with limited teaching and dietitian support. It usually takes our center about an hour to teach a family how to do it. Unlike the ketogenic diet, pre-made products such as baking mixes, candy bars, and shakes are available in many groceries and restaurants. It allows a child to choose items off a menu at a school cafeteria or restaurant, which is nearly impossible on the ketogenic diet. Families can buy *Dr. Atkins' New Diet Revolution* or a carbohydrate gram counter (e.g., *CalorieKing* guides) in almost any bookstore or online nowadays and begin the diet at home. Although less restrictive, there is less dietitian support, so families need to be more independent. Constipation, acidosis, and weight loss seem to be less common, but the two diets have never been studied against each other prospectively to compare. Lastly, parents can do the Atkins diet themselves, along with their child. Even your doctor can do it!

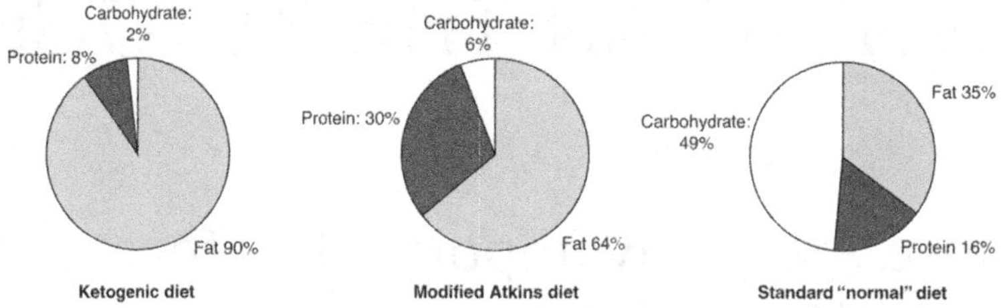

FIGURE 18.1 Compositions of ketogenic, modified Atkins, and standard diets.

WHY IS THERE A NEED FOR ALTERNATIVES?

Other than perhaps the MCT oil diet and availability of Nutricia KetoCal®, the ketogenic diet in use today is remarkably similar to that created 80 years ago.

Do we need something new? Maybe.

We have found the modified Atkins diet to be helpful for children with significant behavioral problems in which the ketogenic diet's restrictiveness would cause problems. Not all epilepsy centers in the world offer the ketogenic diet, as it requires a specially trained dietitian and medical team; the Atkins diet may be a partial solution. Some children have had difficulty with high cholesterol and poor growth; this *may* be less of an issue with a lower ratio (and higher protein) diet. Adolescents and adults, commonly discouraged from trying the ketogenic diet (whether this is right or wrong!), might be the ideal candidates for the modified Atkins diet. Lastly, if it is truly easier to start and stick to, maybe the modified Atkins diet could be used early in the course of seizures, in some cases *before* medications?

TABLE 18.1 Differences Between the Ketogenic Diet and the Modified Atkins Diet

	Ketogenic Diet	Modified Atkins Diet
Calories (% RDA)	Measured carefully	Unrestricted
Fluids	Measured, but often ad lib	Unrestricted
Fat	80%	60%
Protein	15%	30%
Carbohydrates	5%	10%
Fasting period	Occasionally done	No
Admission to hospital	Usually	No
Meal plans computer-created	Yes	No
Foods weighed and measured	Yes	No
Sharing of foods at family meals	No	Yes
Ability to eat foods made in restaurants	No	Yes
"Low carbohydrate" store-bought products	Not used	Allowed sparingly

	Ketogenic Diet	Modified Atkins Diet
Intensive education provided	Yes	No
Multiple studies over many years proving benefits	Yes	Yes, recently

FUTURE DIRECTIONS

The modified Atkins diet is now over 8 years old. It works in 49% of children (and adults) who start it. Over 200 patients have been started just in the medical literature, with likely double that number who haven't been published in any trial. The percentage of patients who it works for is strikingly similar to the ketogenic diet. However, they have never been formally compared in the same study with large numbers as a randomized trial. Although this has been discussed, we are not sure it would sway parents or physicians to use one diet over another no matter what the results were. We see these diets as complementary and not competing.

At Johns Hopkins, we generally advocate the ketogenic diet but are willing to use the modified Atkins diet for local patients who need a diet quickly or clearly do not want the ketogenic diet for various reasons. We use it for teenagers and adults. In our Adult Epilepsy Diet Center, the modified Atkins diet is the diet of choice. Many of our long-term patients on the ketogenic diet for over 10 years are being switched over. For young babies and children, however, we lean toward the ketogenic diet due to both the easy availability of ketogenic diet formulas and the need for more careful monitoring in this age.

Work is underway to get this diet to developing countries in which there is limited dietitian support. Projects are underway in Honduras and parts of China and India. We have discussed its use for emergency outpatient situations (e.g., Doose syndrome with drop seizures) where children should not wait 1–2 months to start the ketogenic diet. As neurologists and oncologists look at dietary treatments for nonepilepsy uses, the modified Atkins diet may be a more reasonable option for potentially years of use than the ketogenic diet if the condition is not perceived to be as serious as epilepsy (e.g., migraines).

CHAPTER NINETEEN

How Do I Use the Modified Atkins Diet?

So far we've talked about the history of the modified Atkins diet (MAD) and future directions, as well as what the diet basically is. In this chapter, we'll give you the "MAD: 101," which is what we do when we counsel our families. Lastly, we'll talk about fine-tuning the MAD and switching from the MAD to the ketogenic diet.

THE BASICS OF THE FIRST MONTH

In general, this is meant to be simple. If it's not, something's wrong! Before starting the MAD (or any diet), make sure your child doesn't have a reason *not* to start a diet—your neurologist will know. Also, get a baseline fasting set of blood work, including a CBC, SMA20 (CMP), and fasting lipid profile. Appendix F lists many of these labs.

We start by telling families that carbohydrates need to be reduced to 10 grams per day (20 grams for adults). We start adolescents at 10 grams per day, but if it's too hard after 1 week, we'll go up to 15. For the MAD, it doesn't matter which carbohydrates you use, although 99% of our patients naturally choose the lower glycemic index carbohydrates because you get "more bang for your buck" in terms of carbohydrates. It is also important not to go *lower* than 10 grams per day: There will be no additional benefit, and it will just make the diet tougher. Food records show that most parents are already within 5 grams of 10 grams/day of carbohydrate when we check—you will do a good job!

Carbohydrate-counting guides are important to show you the contents of most foods out there. In our opinion, the best one is the *CalorieKing* paperback, which is updated each year, includes restaurants, and is about $10 (www.calorieking.com). There are also carbohydrate-content lists of common foods available on the Internet. We list some basic foods from the Atkins books in Appendix C. After a while, you'll get familiar with the contents of most foods your child likes, and you won't need to refer to this book often.

Second, it is important to remember that this is a high fat diet. We will often tell families that foods should "shine" from the flash of a photograph if you take one! The meals should look similar to those on the ketogenic diet. In fact, we give recipes of ketogenic diet foods. KetoCalculator can be used; just calculate a 2:1 ratio to be safe, and double check the number of carbohydrates per day. However, this is usually not needed as meals are flexible and calories are not restricted. Eat typical ketogenic diet foods such as heavy whipping cream, oils, butter, mayonnaise, and soft cheese. On the MAD, these foods are not only ad lib in regards to amounts, but encouraged.

Calories are ad lib. However, just like on the ketogenic diet, we try not to make children gain significant weight. Hunger should not be an issue—if your child is hungry for breakfast, give more eggs! If they are hungry for lunch, give more tuna or hamburger. Just don't forget the fat, which can be very satisfying, so it's probably better to give more butter and oils. Protein is also ad lib, so good sources like meats, fish, and soy can be given as much as your child wants (but again, don't give them at the expense of fats). Fluids are not only ad lib, but we push them. To date we have not seen a kidney stone in a child on the MAD, and that may be due to the extra fluids or less urinary calcium or acid. Drinks such as diet sodas and flavored waters (e.g., Fruit2O®, Aquafina Flavor Splash®, Powerade Zero®, Nestle Pure Life Natural Fruit Flavored Water®, Dasani Natural Flavored Water®, O Clear Water®) are great and really help. Artificial sweeteners are fine. Extra fluids may make the urine seem less ketotic (due to more fluid), but that's okay.

For the first month, check urine ketones as you would on the ketogenic diet using ketostix. During the first month, they will likely be large. You might even see over-ketosis (see Chapter 7). However, in some children they can be lower (e.g., moderate) or fluctuate. In our experience, the larger the ketones the first month the better, so give lots of fat if the ketones seem to be dropping. Check them twice a week, and record them on a monthly calendar, along with seizures. In addition, we recommend checking your child's weight weekly.

Start a low-carbohydrate multivitamin and calcium. Any tablet form is fine, as well as the sugar-free chewables (e.g., Bugs Bunny® or Scooby Doo®). This is as important as it is on the ketogenic diet. We do not use other supplements such as carnitine, selenium, or Polycitra K®, unlike the ketogenic diet in which we often do.

During the first month, we have a "tough love" approach. We do not reduce medications, but similar to the ketogenic diet, we switch to carb-free preparations. We also stick to 10 grams per day (20 grams for adults). One of our studies surprisingly found that 10 grams per day (for a child) was better than 20 grams per day for the first 3 months (we didn't test formally switching earlier at 1 month). Try to avoid carbohydrate-free store products the first month, such as those made by Atkins and other companies. In general, they are fine, but only after the first month. Let's see what the MAD can do by itself without any other changes.

THE INTERNET IS YOUR FRIEND

We give families lots of recipes and ideas. However, most of the information we get is from the Internet. Recipes are available at www.atkins.com and www.myketocal.com. We also list some recipes in Chapter 23 and ideas of what meal plans may look like in Appendix E. It is sometimes easier to tell families what they *can't* eat (e.g., cookies, candies, pasta, rice) than what they *can.* In this way, ideas for foods and recipes can be critical.

Another trick we use is to tell families to go shopping before actually starting the MAD. We often counsel families on Fridays and tell them to fill out a 3-day food record from Friday–Sunday of foods their child is eating already. This gives our dietitians a chance to see what the child's normal intake (especially calories) is, but it also gives the family the weekend to hit the store and shop. Bring your child and let them be part of the shopping.

KETOCAL® : A BOOST TO THE MAD

In 2010, we published results from a study in which we tested our theory that a higher fat version of the MAD would work better. By using KetoCal® as a supplement, parents were able to raise the average ketogenic diet ratio of the MAD from 1:1 (historically) to 1.8:1. This improved the chances of the MAD working to a remarkable 80% (from about 50% without KetoCal®). Although certainly giving more natural fat (or MCT oil) might achieve the same goal, we have found that Keto-

Cal® is a potentially easy and palatable way to sneak in the extra fat.

The other part of this study was to see if this was only important for the first month. This also was true. As shown in other studies, after 1 month you can lighten up on the restrictions of any diet, and the KetoCal® could be stopped. About 1 in 5 children had slight worsening of seizures, but this is typical for anyone on the diet after the first month. Of course, if your child loves the KetoCal®, it can be continued.

In the study, children were given a case (6 cans) of KetoCal® 4:1 powder. This can be purchased from the company and costs about $150. We told families to get in 60 grams per day, which is 2/3 of a cup of the powder. It can be used as a milkshake (mixing with either water or Fruit2O®) or the powder can be used to cook with (recipes at www.myketocal.com). The milkshake is made by mixing 2/3 of a cup of KetoCal® with 8 ounces (240mL) of water to make a 10-ounce shake, which is about 400 calories. Many families reported to us that the milkshakes taste better cold (made the night before) and flavored with either Fruit2O® as the liquid source, carbohydrate-free flavorings (e.g., Bickford®, Starbucks®), or sugar-free Jell-O®. The times to drink it were also up to the family—most children drank the shakes all at once, either for lunch or as an afternoon snack. The carbohydrates in KetoCal® given this way do not need to be counted toward the daily limit.

KetoCal® also comes in a pre-made liquid form now, in small cartons ("tetrapaks") that look like juice boxes. The premade packs were not tested in our study, but there is no reason to think they won't work as well. We would suggest one pack per day, which is pretty close to 400 calories.

After the first month, if your child doesn't like the KetoCal® (or it's too expensive), it definitely can be stopped without losing seizure control. The decision at this point is up to you.

READING THE FOOD LABELS

Food labels are critical for any processed or prepared foods. Remember that the carbohydrate content highlighted on the front of the packaging for many low-carb products can be somewhat misleading, as not only fiber but sugar alcohols are excluded (see later for more on this). Look for the total carbohydrate amount and subtract only fiber. This is the final amount for that product. Remember portions can be your friend, too: If a candy bar has 10 grams of carbohydrate in it, you can have your child only eat half for 5 grams.

MONTH TWO: TIME TO LIGHTEN UP!

Now that you and your child have succeeded in making it to the end of the first month, things can be made less strict if the diet is helping. We do recommend making one change at a time, similar to the ketogenic diet. Each week things can be changed, very carefully, if desired.

The first change that is possible is to increase carbohydrates. Go up by 5 grams of carbohydrate/day each month if desired (e.g., to 15 grams/day for month 2 and 20 grams/day for month 3). For most children, we will not go higher than 20 grams/day and adults to 30 grams/day. Surprisingly, most children are doing well at 10 grams/day, and this switch is not usually the first one to be made.

The second change is to stop the KetoCal®. As this will lower the ratio slightly by itself, compensate by giving more fat if possible. This is a change to the MAD, so if you plan to stop the KetoCal® (as all families did in our study), count this as a change and do not increase carbs, for example, at the same time.

A third possible change is to reduce medications. We are all in favor of giving this a shot, just do it slowly and leave the MAD unchanged if you're going to do this. If seizures worsen, consider increasing the medications back if medically indicated.

A fourth and final change is to start using low carbohydrate products. Remember to read the food labels as discussed earlier. At this point we don't count fiber toward the carbohydrate limit, but we do count sugar alcohols (e.g., xylitol, maltitol), which can be in many candy bars and low-carb baking mixes. Another way to think of it is *fiber is free.* If you choose to use these products, and many of our families do, just try one new one per week to make sure it doesn't make seizures worse. Some favorites include the Atkins candy bars, shitake mushroom noodles, low-carb chocolate milk, and baking mixes. Just the Cheese™ snacks are also a great and crunchy snack.

You can also now be less strict about checking ketones. Our studies have shown that it is natural and normal on the MAD to have large ketosis in the first month but moderate (or trace) ketosis by the sixth month. In most of these children, they were still doing great, or even better. Keep track on the seizure calendar and show your neurologist. We recommend once weekly ketones on the MAD after the first month.

LONG-TERM USE AND MONITORING

After 1 month (or definitely by 3 months) you should be touching base with your neurologist and dietitian. By this point, you should have a good sense if the MAD is helping. If it is, then we recommend filling out a new 3-day food record (now that your child is on the MAD) and rechecking the labs you did before starting the MAD. These results should be compared, especially the total cholesterol and triglycerides. If they are too high, then adjustments to the types of fat may need to be made. Your child should also be seen by the dietitian to check his/her weight and height and answer your questions. Although side effects appear to be less frequent with the MAD compared to the ketogenic diet, they still can occur and need to be looked out for.

FINE-TUNING THE MAD

Unlike the ketogenic diet, there are fewer specific changes that a dietitian can make to the MAD if things are either not going well from the start, or seizure control is lost. This can definitely be a disadvantage to the MAD, but there are some changes that can be made that we have found helpful. Of course, the *ultimate* fine-tuning change is to switch to the ketogenic diet, but that is not usually necessary. More details on that switch are in the next section.

Usually the first thing we do is look at the seizure calendar and see if ketones are high and also if they correlate to seizure control. If there is a correlation and ketones are low, we'll look at a 3-day food record and make sure enough fat is being given. We might also add extra fat sources such as MCT oil or KetoCal® (assuming the latter has been stopped after the first month by the parent). Carnitine has also been helpful for some of our patients. One of the most common mistakes made by parents is to make the MAD a high-protein rather than a high-fat diet.

Secondly, we'll double check the 3-day food record to look at calories. Some children may be eating much less than before the MAD started, and we'll recommend more calories for more fuel, and then more ketones. Surprisingly, others may be eating too many calories. We've recommended to families to take the same foods they've been giving and reduce them by a quarter or third (because we don't strictly calculate calories). Just make sure the calories reduced are protein, not fat.

Lastly, we'll make sure medications are not playing a role (either too little or too much), as discussed in Chapter 12 and Appendix A. Look for hidden carbohydrates too.

SHOULD I SWITCH FROM THE MAD TO THE KETOGENIC DIET?

This is a tough decision. Lots of studies suggest that you can switch your child from the traditional ketogenic diet to the MAD after months or years without loss of seizure control. In fact, this was how we realized this diet worked. Studies show that diets do not need to be so strict after the initial month or two. However, some children can have more seizures with the MAD, similar to those who have more seizures when the ratio is lowered. Just make sure to do this with your neurologist and dietitian's permission. We usually recommend continuing the multivitamin and calcium but stopping the Polycitra K when you switch to the MAD.

What about the reverse? Going from the MAD to the ketogenic diet? This is an even tougher decision. Most families come to us for the MAD, as they don't want to weigh and measure foods, be admitted, and be able to order out at restaurants. The ketogenic diet is a higher level of work for sure. A recent study from our center in combination with those in Germany, South Korea, and Denmark found that 37% of children who make the switch will have at least a 10% improvement in seizures. Only a few became seizure free, though; interestingly, it was those with Doose syndrome. No child who didn't improve with the MAD then improved at all with the ketogenic diet, although since this study, we have heard of children improving at other hospitals.

What does this tell us about both diets? It suggests that these diets are more alike than different, and the ketogenic diet is probably just a "higher dose" of dietary therapy than the MAD. It also tells us that although the MAD is often excellent for Doose syndrome, if your child is not seizure free after about 6 months, you may want to strongly consider switching to the ketogenic diet.

Discontinuing the modified Atkins diet

In general, we slowly taper the diet until ketones are lost, similar to the ketogenic diet. Go up by 10 grams of carbohydrate per day every 2 weeks until your child reaches 60 grams/day. If seizures worsen, pause and let your neurologist and dietitian know. Once most children reach 60 grams/day they will start to see periods with no ketosis in the urine. Be careful as the MAD may still be working—this is not that different at this point than the low-glycemic index treatment. We'll then tell families to make big substitutions of protein sources for fat (e.g., more tuna than mayonnaise, and more egg than butter/oil as opposed to vice versa).

After 2 weeks of this, you can start switching daily meals each week, one at a time, for more "regular" meals. For example, for 1 week, give a lunch with bread, lots of fruit, and not high fat or protein. The next week, give both lunch *and* breakfast this way. The third and final week, your child will be off the diet. Most families will wait to give high sugar snacks (e.g., cookies, chocolate, pasta) until this point. Some may never give these snacks again!

FREQUENTLY ASKED QUESTIONS

1. *Do I need a dietitian or neurologist?*

   Yes. Preferably both, but at least one. This is a medical diet and needs supervision for side effects, efficacy, medication adjustment, weight gain and health, and so forth. We have received many emails from families who have started the diet on their own: Some have done well, but many have not. Even the ones who have done well usually have many questions that should be answered by a ketoteam.

2. *Do I have to use KetoCal®?*

   Definitely not. However, it's a nice, convenient way to get the extra fat in during the first month of the MAD. You can use MCT oil, heavy whipping cream, or other sources of fat instead if you want.

3. *What materials do I need to start the MAD?*

   This book is a great start. There's also good information on the Internet, including recipes. Many centers also provide printed materials including recipes, seizure calendars, blank food records. In addition, a carb-counting guide (e.g., *CalorieKing)* can be very helpful.

4. *How long before I know if it's helping?*

   Similar to the ketogenic diet, usually the MAD works quickly—within 2–4 weeks. However, a lot depends upon the seizure frequency when you start. For example, if seizures are every 2 months, you may need 6–9 months to know if there has been a true decrease. We usually tell families to give the MAD (or Ketogenic diet) 3–6 months.

5. *How often should I check labs?*

   Probably at 3 months and 6 months, then every 6 months after that.

CHAPTER TWENTY

The MCT Ketogenic Diet

This chapter was written by Elizabeth Neal RD, PhD. Based in the United Kingdom, Dr. Neal is a world expert in the MCT diet.

By the mid-20th century, when the classic ketogenic diet was falling out of favor because of availability of new anticonvulsants and a feeling that large amounts of fat were unpalatable, Dr. Peter Huttenlocher of the University of Chicago set out to invent a new and improved form of ketogenic diet. He believed that the ketogenic diet was an effective form of therapy and that more families would try—and benefit from—a ketogenic diet if it were formulated with foods more closely approximating a normal diet. Dr. Huttenlocher and his group replaced some of the long chain fat in the classic ketogenic diet; that, is fat from foods such as butter, oils, cream, and mayonnaise, with an alternative fat source with a shorter carbon chain length. This medium chain fat, otherwise known as medium chain triglyceride (MCT), is absorbed more efficiently than long chain fat, is carried directly to the liver in the portal blood, and does not require carnitine to transport it into cell mitochondria for oxidation. These metabolic differences give MCT increased ketogenic potential, that is, it will yield more ketones per kilocalorie of energy provided than its long chain counterparts. This increased ketogenic potential means less total fat is needed in the MCT diet. Whereas the classical 4:1 ratio ketogenic diet provides 90% of its calories from fat, the MCT ketogenic diet typically provides 70–75% energy from fat (both MCT and long chain), allowing more protein and carbohydrate foods to be included. The increased carbohydrate and protein allowance makes the MCT diet a useful option for some children, especially those with limited food choices.

The original MCT diet provided 60% of energy from MCT; the remaining 40% was usually divided up to provide 10% energy from protein, 15–19% energy from carbohydrate, and 11–15% from long chain fat. However, this level of MCT can cause gastrointestinal discomfort in some children, such as abdominal cramps, diarrhea, and vomiting, especially if the MCT is introduced too quickly into the diet. For this reason, Schwartz et al. in 1989 suggested using a modified MCT diet, which reduced the calories from MCT to 30% of total and added an extra 30% of calories from chain fat. In many children, this lower amount of MCT may not be enough to ensure adequate ketosis for optimal seizure control, and in practice, a starting MCT level somewhere between the two (40–50% energy) is likely to be the best balance between gastrointestinal tolerance and good ketosis. This can then be increased or decreased as necessary during fine-tuning.

Schwartz and her group also compared the clinical and metabolic effects of the MCT ketogenic diet, both traditional (60% MCT) and modified (30% MCT), with the classical 4:1 ketogenic diet. They found all three diets equally effective in controlling seizures, but compliance and palatability were better with the classic/ketogenic diet. However, in this study children were not randomly allocated to one of the diets, leaving it open to possibility of bias. The question of differences in efficacy and tolerability between the classic and MCT ketogenic diets was looked at again by Neal et al. in 2009, but this time using a randomized study design. One hundred forty-five children with intractable epilepsy were randomized to receive a classic or MCT diet. Seizure frequency was assessed after 3, 6, and 12 months, and these data were available for analysis from 94 children: 45 on a classic diet and 49 on a MCT diet. Table 20.1 shows results for percentage of baseline seizure frequency between the two groups after 3, 6, and 12 months Although the mean value was lower in the classic group after 6 and 12 months, these differences were not statistically significant at any of the times (the *P* value is greater than 0.05 at 3, 6, and 12 months). There were also no significant differences in numbers achieving greater than 50% or 90% seizure reduction. Serum acetoacetate and ß-hydroxybutyrate levels at 3 and 6 months were significantly higher in children on the classic diet; this was also the case at 12 months for acetoacetate. There were no significant differences in tolerability except increased reports in the classic group of lack of energy after 3 months and vomiting after 12 months. This study concluded that both classic and MCT ketogenic diets have their place in the treatment of childhood epilepsy.

TABLE 20.1 Mean Percentage of Baseline Seizure Numbers at 3, 6, and 12 Months in Classic and MCT Diet Groups

Time (Months)	Classical Diet	MCT Diet	P Value
3	67% (n=45)	69% (n=49)	0.834
6	49% (n=30)	68% (n=34)	0.165
12	41% (n=22)	53% (n=25)	0.382

(n=number providing seizure data at that time point)

So how does the MCT diet work in practice? The MCT is given in the diet as a commercially available MCT oil or emulsion (Liquigen®, SHS in Europe). Both are available by prescription in the United Kingdom. The amount of MCT has to be calculated into the diet just like any other fat and should be divided up over the day and included in all meals and snacks; the amount will be specified in the diet prescription provided by the dietician. Liquigen® can be mixed with milk for an MCT milk drink (best with skimmed or semi-skimmed milk as full fat milk causes the mixture to thicken excessively); it can also be added to foods such as soups and mashed potato, or used in recipes, ranging from sugar-free jelly, sauces, and baking. MCT oil also works well in meal preparation and baking, A number of recipes are available from the Matthew's Friends Web site (www.matthewsfriends.org), which give ideas for MCT meals and snacks. *MCT has a low flashpoint, so be cautious when frying, and keep the temperature fairly low!*

Because the diet allows more carbohydrate and protein, a child on the MCT diet can eat a wider variety of other, antiketogenic foods. Protein portions are more generous than with the classic diet, as are the allowed amounts of fruit and vegetables. Small amounts of higher carbohydrate foods, such as bread, potatoes and cereals, can also be calculated into the daily allowance. As with the classic diet, sweet and sugary foods are not allowed, and calories will still be controlled. Although exact recipes can be calculated for the MCT, many centers will instead use food exchange lists because of the more generous amounts of carbohydrate and protein. The use of separate carbohydrate, protein, and fat exchanges is recommended because this allows an even macronutrient distribution over the meals and snacks. As with the classic ketogenic diet, full vitamin, mineral, and trace element supplementation must be given. The prescribed diet must also meet essential fatty acid requirements.

The MCT diet can be provided as a tube feed for children who need it, but there is not one complete product available as there is for the classic diet, so the prescription and the preparation of such a feed will be much more complicated. For this reason, use of the classic ketogenic diet feed products is preferable.

On commencing the MCT diet, the Liquigen® or MCT oil needs to be introduced much more slowly than long chain fat (over about 5–10 days), as it may cause abdominal discomfort, vomiting, or diarrhea if introduced rapidly. During this introduction period the rest of the diet can be given as prescribed, but an extra meal may be needed to make up the calories while using less MCT. Once on the full diet, children must stick with it just as rigidly as with the classic diet. Fine-tuning is usually needed to maximize benefit and tolerance. This is done by increasing or decreasing the amount of calories provided by MCT; the amount of long chain fat can be adjusted to keep the same total calories from fat in the diet. If a higher level of ketosis is desired and an increased amount of MCT is not tolerated, the amount of carbohydrate in the diet can be reduced and long chain fat increased to balance calories.

Discontinuing the MCT diet should be done in a stepwise process. The amount of MCT fat should be slowly reduced, and the protein and carbohydrate increased. However, if the MCT diet works, as with the classic diet, children stay on it for about 2 years.

MCT oil in small amounts can also be used as a supplement to the classic ketogenic diet, both because it can increase ketosis and because it may decrease the constipation that often accompanies this diet. Swapping some of the long chain fat allowance for MCT can soften the stools of constipated children and in small amounts is well tolerated.

CHAPTER TWENTY ONE

The LGIT (Low Glycemic Index Treatment)

This chapter was written by Heidi H. Pfeifer, RD, LDN, the ketogenic dietitian at Massachusetts General Hospital in Boston and co-creator of the LGIT diet.

The Low Glycemic Index Treatment (LGIT) for epilepsy was developed in 2002 at the Massachusetts General Hospital by dietitian Heidi Pfeifer and Dr. Elizabeth Thiele as a liberalized alternative to the ketogenic diet. Although effective, the ketogenic diet can be difficult to tolerate due to restrictiveness and poor palatability. To meet the therapeutic ketogenic ratio (4:1 fats to protein and carbohydrates), fats must comprise an extremely high percentage of the daily caloric intake (90%). However, the LGIT is lower in fat (60%) and higher in carbohydrates with a therapeutic ratio that is closer to 1:1. The modified Atkins diet approximates a 2:1 ratio.

The concept of low glycemic index treatment is new to the field of neurology. However, similar therapies have been used over the past 20 years for diabetes, heart disease, obesity, and polycystic ovary syndrome. A specific food's glycemic index refers to its effect on blood sugar level as compared to a reference food, like sugar. A number of different variables, such as acidity or fiber levels, can affect a food's glycemic index; for a given food, the higher these levels, the lower the glycemic index. The glycemic index can be modified by adding fats or proteins to carbohydrates, slowing digestion, and, therefore, lowering the glycemic index. For example, adding butter to bread lowers its glycemic index. A sample of common glycemic index values is listed in Table 21.1. More detail can be found on the Internet (www .glycemicindex.com)

The LGIT is similar to the modified Atkins diet and ketogenic diet as it regulates the quantity of carbohydrates consumed, typically to 40–60 grams per day. A main difference compared to the modified Atkins diet and ketogenic diet is that other than the higher carbohydrate count per day, carbohydrate-rich foods are limited to those with a glycemic index of <50 relative to glucose. On the modified Atkins diet, the type of carbohydrate is not specified, although with only 10–20 grams per day, most patients may tend to gravitate toward the lower glycemic index carbs naturally.

TABLE 21.1 Glycemic Index of Common Foods (Those Foods Under 50 Are Highlighted in Grey)

Food	Glycemic Index
Lettuce	10
Peanuts	15
Broccoli	15
Eggplant	15
Tomatoes	15

Food	Glycemic Index
Soy beans	16
Pears	38
Apples	38
Peaches	42
Grapes	46
Popcorn	55
Cheese pizza	60
Ice cream	61
Raisins	64
Pineapple	66
Mashed potato	70
Waffles	76
Donut	76
Pretzels	83
Baked potato	85
Dates	103

Like the ketogenic diet, the LGIT is individualized to each patient's needs. Goals for protein, fat, and carbohydrate intake are provided before treatment initiation to ensure that each patient's diet meets his or her nutritional needs. However, unlike the ketogenic diet, the LGIT does not require foods to be weighed, as meals are based on every-day portion sizes. This allows family members to eat similar foods at mealtime, as well as to eat together in restaurants while maintaining treatment compliance. Compared to the ketogenic and modified Atkins diets, there is less fat with the LGIT, but many of the foods do end up having fats in them for satiety.

Breakfast

Scrambled egg—2 eggs, 1 oz cheese, 1tsp butter
Peach
Heavy cream—2oz

Lunch

Roast beef sandwich
Low-carb pita pocket—1/2
Roast beef—4oz
Cheddar cheese—1oz
Horseradish mayonnaise—1/2tbsp
Roasted red pepper—1/2 cup
Heavy cream—2oz

Snack

Cheese stick—1
Apple—1/2

Dinner

Grilled chicken salad
Chicken breast—6oz
Mixed salad with lettuce, tomato, and cucumber
Heavy cream—2oz
Blue cheese dressing—1tbsp

Although less restrictive, the efficacy of the LGIT is similar to that of the ketogenic diet. Recent studies demonstrate that more than half of patients on the LGIT achieve >50% reduction in their seizure activity with some patients achieving seizure freedom. Many patients have also been able to reduce their anticonvulsant medications while on the LGIT. Treatment has proven effective for both generalized and partial onset seizures and for an age range from 2 years through adulthood.

Patients on the LGIT are monitored very closely and, at our center, are seen by a dietitian and a neurologist 1 month after initiating the diet and then at 3-month intervals throughout therapy. During appointments, clinicians assess seizure control, measure height and weight, and obtain labs to monitor for side effects. With this information, the dietitian and neurologist can make necessary adjustments to optimize the LGIT.

No severe side effects have been reported in patients on the LGIT. Minor possible side effects include weight loss, acidosis, and constipation. Those individuals who have experienced weight loss often did so intentionally. Patients with symptoms of acidosis experienced lethargy, nausea, vomiting, and headache. However, acidosis can be monitored with a simple blood test and easily treated with an alkalizing agent. Just as on the ketogenic diet, constipation is an issue but is minimized on the LGIT by a higher fiber intake in combination with optimal fluids.

The therapeutic mechanism of the LGIT remains unknown. However, we do know that the diet alters metabolism with fats used as the primary source of energy instead of carbohydrates. This reduction in glycolytic stress is thought to contribute to the therapeutic mechanism of dietary treatment. Fat metabolism results in the production of ketone bodies. In LGIT, the ketone bodies may be present in the blood or urine at lower levels than seen in the ketogenic diet and may be undetectable. Additionally, the stabilization of glucose levels may provide a therapeutic effect. Studies have demonstrated a positive correlation between over 90% seizure control and lower blood glucose levels.

As with any other seizure therapy, when seizure freedom is achieved, the patient may slowly transition off treatment. In the case of LGIT, larger quantities of carbohydrates with a low glycemic index (GI <50) are slowly introduced into the diet. If seizure freedom is not achieved, the patient, family, and clinicians need to assess the benefits of current dietary therapy, as well as discuss other possible treatment options to determine future care.

KEY POINTS TO MAKING THE LGIT A SUCCESS

- Always balance each meal with a protein source, a fat source, and a carbohydrate source.

- Limit daily carbohydrate intake to 40–60 grams spread evenly throughout the day.
- Use carbohydrate foods that have glycemic index values that are less than 50.
- Increase the amount of protein (chicken, fish, beef, eggs, cheese, tofu, etc.) and fats (butter, oil, margarine, and mayonnaise).
- Transition from milk to cream to decrease the amount of carbohydrates that are consumed.
- Provide appropriate vitamin and mineral supplements to meet individual needs in the setting of decreased carbohydrate intake.
- Ensure close follow up with a dietitian and neurologist well versed in dietary treatment of epilepsy. ALL DIETS need to be done with the help of a ketogenic team!

SECTION V

Ketogenic Cooking

CHAPTER TWENTY TWO

Sample Meal Plans for the Ketogenic Diet

Although quantities are limited and smaller than a child is used to, the variety and appeal of food on the ketogenic diet are limited only by your creativity!

- Filet of beef with strawberry cream popsicle
- Chicken teriyaki lettuce wraps
- Eggs Benedict
- Cheese omelet with bacon
- Shrimp scampi with pumpkin parfait
- Cheesecake

Nearly all the foods your child likes can be transformed into a ketogenic meal. The ketogenic diet can be such a gift—the meals need not be considered a punishment.

> *AS OFTEN AS POSSIBLE, Michael has something that we are having. If I am making pork chops for us, I cook him one. If we are having tuna fish sandwiches, he has tuna fish with mayonnaise wrapped in a leaf of lettuce.*

Parents should not stray from the basic meal plans in the beginning for the sake of simplicity and control while learning how to implement the diet and seeing whether ketosis provides effective seizure control for their child. When the diet has been proven useful and they are familiar with its preparation, parents can begin to get more creative with new food items and new menu plans.

Herbs and spices, lemon juice, soy sauce, baking chocolate, ketchup, and other flavorings all contain carbohydrates. The overall carbohydrate level in the diet is extremely low so that ketchup calculated into a meal plan may decrease your child's fruit or vegetable allotment! Herbs and spices should be limited to a pinch, and high-carbohydrate flavorings such as ketchup or chocolate should only be used occasionally, if at all.

Pure extracts, like vanilla or strawberry, are allowed up to five drops a meal and can be considered "free," which is to say not affecting the ketogenic balance of the meal. Other pure, carbohydrate-free extracts, such as almond, lemon, or chocolate, are similarly free. Some children do not even like the taste of the extracts, and they are not essential for the diet but are there to add flavoring to some foods.

> *IT WAS IMPORTANT TO MY SON to feel as though he was getting a dessert. So I always kept a stock of homemade cream popsicles in the freezer, flavored with vanilla or chocolate (which was calculated into his meal plans) and a little bit of saccharin. He got one after every dinner. If he was supposed to have 80cc of cream and the Tupperware popsicle molds only held 60cc, he drank the rest of the cream straight.*

Think of the recipes included in this chapter in terms of entire meal plans, not as single food items. The ketogenic ratio of food in the diet must balance within a whole meal, so any food calculated into one part of the meal affects what can go into other parts. All the ingredients in the meal can be baked or cooked together, or each item can be eaten separately to equal the correct calories and ratio.

The menus that follow are examples drawn from the experience of various parents and are for a "generic" child. Your own meal plans will take into account your child's calorie level, protein needs, ketogenic ratio, and individual preferences.

> *GO TO RESTAURANTS! Eat together as a family. Enjoy the benefits you get from the diet. Try not to segregate your child or feed her separately from the rest of the family. She will enjoy feeling included. Most kids appreciate the reduction of seizures and freedom from medication more than they covet the food they cannot eat.*

TIPS

Following are tips from parents who have experienced the ketogenic diet:

- Kids don't mind eating the same thing over and over. Find several simple menus that you and your child can agree on, and stick with them. Six to eight menus is probably all you'll need. The multivitamin and calcium will take care of the rest.

- Use a salad or dessert plate and bowl so the amount of food does not appear small.
- Fix a few meals in advance and keep them in the refrigerator in carefully labeled Tupperware containers in case you are not there at mealtimes, or for when your child goes to school or to a friend's house. You will build up a huge Tupperware collection.
- Use the pinch of spices that are allowed (but remember they do contain carbohydrate). A small amount goes a long way toward making the food interesting.
- My son will drink the cream straight down, but I often mix it with sugar-free soda so it will fill him up more.
- Save a couple of favorite meals for extra special times. Use these meals less than once a week so they remain special for times when you are having something your child loves but cannot have, or for times when nothing else sounds good.
- Chopped lettuce with mayonnaise can be a fairly large-looking element of a meal. It really helps fill up the plate, and it helps with bowel movements.
- Find places to hide the fat. Oil hides well in applesauce or ice cream. Butter disappears into peanut butter or cream cheese. Tuna, chicken, or egg salad eats up mayonnaise.
- Select dishes that are familiar and resemble your family's normal meals.

- Don't assume that a zero-calorie powdered drink is OK. Some contain hidden sources of carbohydrates and may say on the label "when prepared this drink will provide 5 calories."
- Don't mix medicine or supplements that have a bad taste with food. Separate medicines from food as much as possible. Sometimes sprinkles of medicines can be mixed in as long as your child can't taste it.
- Do not buy diet foods—use real mayonnaise, butter, eggs, and so on. Diet foods tend to have high water content and extra carbohydrates.
- Counter the small quantity of food with creative shapes and arrangements: Slice meat thinly and fan it out. Pound chicken paper-thin. Cut carrots into carrot chips, cucumbers into shoestring sticks.

BASIC TECHNIQUES

The recipes in this chapter do not have quantities, as these must be calculated for each individual child. Each recipe is for a whole meal, considered as a unit, because foods in one part of the meal affect what can be included in another part while maintaining the prescribed ketogenic ratio. As a rule, ingredients such as catsup, lemon juice, vinegar, herbs and spices, soy sauce, and baking chocolate are used in very small quantities (such as 2 grams, about 1/8 teaspoon).

Meats should be lean with fat removed. Fish and poultry should be skinless and boneless. This is to ensure that the child's protein allotment will be as close to pure or solid protein as possible.

Cooked foods should be trimmed and weighed on the gram scale after cooking, except in the case of food that is heated only slightly or will not change volume during cooking (such as cheese for melting or eggs). Previously cooked foods do not have to be weighed again after reheating.

The following exchange lists show whether a specific vegetable should be weighed raw or cooked. "What the eye sees, the mind remembers," the old adage goes. But food amounts should not be "guesstimated." You may get used to judging how much 25 grams of chicken or 15 grams of applesauce is, but you should always check with a scale for accuracy. The quantity of each ingredient in these menus varies from child to child, so we have not given exact amounts here. Quantities can be calculated either by hand or by using a computer program in consultation with a doctor or dietitian.

EXCHANGE LISTS

In the hand-calculated ketogenic diet, fruits and vegetables with similar carbohydrate contents have been grouped into lists of items that may be substituted for one another interchangeably (Table 22.1). This also assumes to some degree that you're not using a computer program like KetoCalculator. We include this in this edition mostly for your own knowledge and historical purposes. In general, Group A vegetables have half the carbohydrates of Group B, so you are allowed more.

When a menu calls for 21 grams of 10% fruit, you may choose cantaloupe, orange, strawberry, peach, or any other item from the 10% fruit list. Or you may choose to use 14 grams (two-thirds the amount prescribed) of a 15% fruit, such as blueberries, pear, or pineapple. Similarly, if a menu calls for 18 grams of a Group B vegetable, you may choose any item or combination of items from the Group B list, including broccoli, mushrooms, or green beans. Or you may choose to use twice that amount, 36 grams, of any Group A vegetable or combination of Group A vegetables, including asparagus, celery, and summer squash.

All the other ingredients in the diet, including meats, fats, and cheeses, should be specified individually in each menu.

Exchange lists allow greater flexibility in using fruits and vegetables. The diet works well with this method, in spite of minor variations in the makeup of each vegetable and fruit. If a child is eating exclusively high-carbohydrate fruits and vegetables such as grapes and carrots, menus should be calculated specifically for these items.

When hand calculation was the norm, meats, fats, and cheeses were also used in generic exchange list form. In spite of significant variations in the content of items on each exchange list, this worked well for some children who could tolerate the resulting fluctuation in diet content. In an effort to provide optimal ketosis for the greatest number of children, and with the more precise computer menu planning now the norm, only fruit and vegetables are now used in generic exchange list form.

TABLE 22.1

Exchange Lists

Fruit: Fresh or Canned Without Sugar

10%		15%	
(Use amount prescribed)		(Use 2/3 amount prescribed)	
Applesauce, Mott's	Papaya	Apple	Kiwi
Cantaloupe	Peach	Apricot	Mango
Grapefruit	Strawberries	Blackberries	Nectarine
Grapes, purple	Tangerine	Blueberries	Pear
Honeydew melon	Watermelon	Figs	Pineapple
Orange	Grapes, green	Raspberries	

Vegetables: Fresh, Canned, or Frozen
Measure raw (R) or cooked (C) as specified

Group A Vegetables		Group B Vegetables	
(Use twice amount prescribed)		(Use amount prescribed)	
Asparagus/C	Radish/R	Beets/C	Kohlrabi/C
Beet greens/C	Rhubarb/R	Broccoli/C	Mushroom/R
Cabbage/C	Sauerkraut/C	Brussels sprouts/C	Mustard greens/C
Celery/C or R	Summer squash/C	Cabbage/R	Okra/C
Chicory/R	Swiss chard/C	Carrots/R or C	Onion/R or C
Cucumbers/R	Tomato/R	Cauliflower/C	Rutabaga/C
Eggplant/C	Tomato juice	Collards/C	Spinach/C
Endive/R	Turnips/C	Dandelion greens/C	Tomato/C
Green pepper/ R or C	Turnip greens/C	Green beans/C	Winter squash/C
Poke/C	Watercress/R	Kale/C	

Fat
Unsaturated fats are recommended

Butter	Canola oil	Flaxseed oil	Margarine
Corn oil	Peanut oil	Mayonnaise	Olive oil

"FREE" WAYS TO DRESS UP YOUR CREAM

Ice cream ball

• Dust with a speck of cinnamon or nutmeg

	• Flavor with sweetener and vanilla or calculated baking chocolate
	• Whip in canola oil after 1 hour of freezing
	• Flavor with sweetener and vanilla or calculated baking chocolate
Whipped parfait	• Layer with calculated berries
	• Sprinkle with a chopped nut
	• Flavor with sweetener and vanilla, lemon, maple, almond, or
	• Serve on top of calculated sugar-free Jell-O
Cream soda	• Pour cream into fruit-flavored sugar-free soda

Note: The following meal plans must be prepared using the calculated food amount specified for an individual child.

DON'T FORGET SUPPLEMENTS. The ketogenic diet must be supplemented with a sugarless multivitamin/mineral and a calcium supplement every day!

SCRAMBLED EGG BREAKFAST

Eggs
Nonstick vegetable oil spray
Butter
Cream
Mandarin oranges

Options (The following must be calculated into the meal plan if desired)

Crisp bacon, ham, or sausage
Grated cheese in omelets
Vegetables, fresh fruit, or applesauce instead of juice
Baking chocolate for cocoa in cream

Beat equal amounts of yolk and white. Cook eggs in a microwave or nonstick pan, which may be sprayed with nonstick vegetable oil. Transfer to scale and weigh, trimming if necessary. Transfer to plate and add any additional butter. For omelets, egg should be cooked flat and thin, then put back in pan, filled with calculated cheese or vegetable/butter mixture, heated slightly, and scraped thoroughly onto a plate with a small rubber spatula. Garnish plate with calculated crisp bacon and/or grated cheese sprinkles.

Dilute cream with water or ice to make it more like milk, or make hot chocolate by melting baking chocolate shavings in cream with sweetener.

Your child must consume all the butter on the plate. Drink orange juice or eat fruit last for dessert. If you choose to include bacon or cheese, less egg will be allowed in the meal plan because the protein allotment will be shared.

KETO PANCAKES WITH "SYRUP"

Egg
Cottage cheese
Sugar-free sweetener
Nonstick vegetable oil spray
Butter
Carbohydrate-free pure maple flavoring
Fresh fruit slices

Beat egg white until stiff. Fold in yolk, cottage cheese, and sweetener. Spray nonstick pan with cooking spray. Pour mixture into pan to form a round disk about 3/4 inch thick. Cook thoroughly on first side before turning (or the pancake will fall apart). Top with "syrup" made of melted butter mixed with a few drops of sweetener and carbohydrate-free pure maple flavoring. Serve with fruit slices on the side.

WESTERN OMELET

Egg
Cream
Nonstick vegetable oil spray
Green pepper
Tomato
Onion
Dill, basil, salt, pepper
Mayonnaise

Scramble egg and weigh. Add a little of allotted cream and scramble again. Pour into heated pan coated with vegetable cooking spray. Chop vegetables. Sprinkle with pinch of spices. Mix with mayonnaise. Spread vegetable/mayonnaise mixture on egg. Then flip top over to make omelet and cook a few more minutes until done. This omelet may also be made in a sandwich machine by pouring half of the egg on the grid, spreading the vegetable mixture on top, then adding the other half of the egg and closing the machine until done.

EASY APPLE-SAUSAGE BAKE

Unsweetened applesauce
Butter
Sugar-free sweetener, vanilla
Bob Evans sausage link
Cream
Speck of cinnamon

Broil sausage link under medium flame until brown, boil until done, or sauté in frying pan. Drain on paper towel. Weigh and trim. Meanwhile, place applesauce in small ovenproof container. Mix in brown sugar substitute or sweetener, top with butter, and place under broiler. Whip cream until it thickens, add a few drops of vanilla and sweetener, and continue beating until stiff. When applesauce is warm and butter is melted, top with whipped cream and dust with cinnamon and serve with the cooked sausage.

APPLESAUCE is a great place to hide fat. As much as equal parts fat to applesauce will blend in and taste good. Add 1/4 grain of saccharin dissolved in warm water or a dash of liquid sweetener to unsweetened applesauce and dust with a speck of cinnamon before serving. May be served warm or at room temperature.

PEANUT BUTTER MUFFINS

4:1 120 calories per 3 muffins
9gm egg,
8gm butter,
4gm Skippy peanut butter

Whip whites until stiff, add yolk, measure 9gms. Melt butter and peanut butter in microwave, and add to egg. Bake 325° for 10–15 minutes. Makes 3 muffins.

KETO COOKIES AND KETO CEREAL (1 SERVING=2 COOKIES)

2 egg whites
1tsp. cream of tartar
Small pkg. sugar-free Jell-O

Beat whites stiff, add tartar and Jell-O, put on nonstick pan, Bake 325°. Bake 6–8min or till brown. Makes 20 cookies. 1 serving=2 cookies.

Keto Cereal can be made by adding coloring to the cookies before baking and crumbling the cookies to make cereal. Serve with allotted cream.

PEANUT BUTTER SANDWICH MEAL

4:1 345 calories
27g egg white
1/4tsp cream of tartar
4g Skippy peanut butter
26g butter
Sugar-free sweetener

Whip egg whites until peaks form. Add cottage cheese, cream of tartar, and a couple drops of sweetener. Plop two piles onto cookie sheet sprayed with Pam nonstick vegetable oil. Bake at 350° for 20–25 minutes (until lightly brown).

To make Bagels, make holes in the middle of the piles before baking. You also can fry these on a griddle; they keep nicely in the fridge. Mix butter and peanut butter together and spread on the "bagel".

STRAWBERRY CHOCOLATE CHIP ICE CREAM WITH BACON

Sugar-free sweetener
Cream
Vanilla
Baking chocolate
Strawberries (or peaches, or raspberries)
Canola oil
Crisp bacon

Ice cream can be made up to a week beforehand. Dissolve saccharin tablet in 1/2 teaspoon of warm water. Add to cream in a small Pyrex dish. Flavor with vanilla to taste, baking chocolate shavings, and sliced fresh strawberries. Freeze about 1 hour, or until ice begins to form. Remove from freezer. Stir in canola oil quickly and return to freezer. Unmold and serve in a small bowl with crisp bacon on the side.

VARY THE FRUIT (peach, raspberry), omit the chocolate or melt it into cream, or add pure maple extract and chopped nuts for variety. Omitting chocolate or substituting chopped nuts for fruit has to be calculated, of course. Cream may be whipped before freezing.

QUICHE LORRAINE (CUSTARD WITH BACON)

Cream
Egg
Bacon
Orange slices

Heat cream to scald. Do not boil. Stir beaten egg into cream. Stir in crumbled bacon. Pour mixture into a custard cup. Place in a pan of water. Microwave or bake at 350° until done (about 25 minutes, or until a silver knife inserted in the middle comes out clean). Serve in the custard cup in the middle of a small plate with thin orange slices arranged around the cup in the shape of a flower.

TUNA SALAD PLATE

Tuna
Celery
Mayonnaise
Sour cream
Parmesan cheese
Lettuce
Cucumber
Tomatoes
Sugar-free Jell-O
Sugar-free sweetener

Cream
Vanilla
Baking chocolate

Mix mayonnaise, celery, and tuna; arrange in center of plate. Stir together sour cream and parmesan; mix with chopped lettuce and arrange around tuna. Garnish plate with cucumbers and tomatoes.

For dessert, sugar-free Jell-O topped with sweetened vanilla whipped cream, sprinkled with baking chocolate shavings.

Options: Hard-boiled egg, cubed chicken or turkey, or baby shrimps may be substituted for the tuna. These salads are easy to prepare in advance, making them ideal travel or school meals.

PEANUT BUTTER CELERY SNACKS

Celery
Peanut butter
Butter

Wash thin celery ribs. Peel to remove any strings. Slice off bottom for better stability. Weigh and trim. Combine peanut butter with half of allotted butter. Mix thoroughly. Fill the cavity of celery ribs with peanut butter-butter mixture. Cut into 3-inch pieces. Note: this menu does not have enough protein to be used as a full meal.

IN THE ABSENCE OF TOAST, it's nice to have something crispy that holds a shape, like celery or cucumber boats.

CHEF'S SALAD WITH MAPLE WALNUT WHIP

Lettuce
Mushrooms
Carrots
Tomato
Cucumber
Olive
American cheese
Ham and/or turkey
Olive oil
Vinegar
Salt, pepper, oregano
(Mayonnaise is optional)
Dried parsley
Accent
Cream
Pure maple extract
Sugar-free sweetener
Crushed walnuts

Combine chopped lettuce, sliced mushrooms, and carrots in a bowl. Arrange tomato and cucumber slices, olive, and strips of cheese, ham, and/or turkey on top. Shake or beat with a fork the oil and vinegar, a speck of salt and pepper, and a few flakes of oregano in a jar with a tight lid (mayonnaise may be substituted for some of the oil for thicker consistency). Pour over salad. Sprinkle a few parsley flakes and a dash of Accent over all.

For dessert: Whip cream until thick. Add 3 or 4 drops of pure maple extract and a few drops of sweetener, and continue whipping until stiff. (Several grams vegetable oil may also be whipped into cream if there is too much oil for the salad.) Heap into a parfait dish. Sprinkle with crushed walnuts and serve.

Optional: To make Butterscotch Fluff instead of Maple Walnut Whip, substitute butterscotch extract instead of maple extract and chopped pecans instead of chopped walnuts.

SPINACH SALAD

Spinach
Red onion
Mushroom
Carrot
Olive oil
Vinegar
Dried mustard
Garlic salt
Pepper

Crisp bacon
Hard-boiled egg
Cream
Vanilla
Sugar-free sweetener

Wash spinach, chop coarsely, place in bowl. Sprinkle with chopped red onion, sliced mushroom, and carrot. Shake oil and vinegar together in a jar with a speck of dried mustard, garlic salt, and pepper. Pour over salad. Sprinkle with crumbled crisp bacon and chopped egg (equal parts white and yolk). Dessert: Serve with vanilla shake or popsicle.

AT ONE POINT MY SON STARTED GAINING TOO MUCH WEIGHT, and I couldn't figure out why. Then Mrs. Kelly and I reviewed everything I was doing. I had started hiding a lot of fat in ice cream in the form of canola oil because my son had gotten tired of eating so much butter on top of everything. But I was measuring the oil, like the cream and juice, by volume. Lighter liquids are approximately equal when measured either by weight or volume. But because it is so heavy, oil has to be measured on a gram scale. When I started measuring the canola oil on the gram scale instead of in the graduated cylinder, the weight gain stopped.

DEVILED EGG WITH BERRY PARFAIT

Hard-boiled egg
Butter, mayonnaise
Carrots, celery, onion
Dried mustard, paprika
Lettuce
Strawberries or raspberries
Grated lemon rind
Cream, vanilla, sweetener, chocolate

Cut egg in half lengthwise and weigh equal amounts of white and yolk. Mix yolk thoroughly with mayonnaise, a few grams melted butter, a speck of dried mustard, chopped celery, and onion. Spoon yolk mixture back into the egg white. Sprinkle with salt and pepper.

Dust with paprika. Serve on a plate with chopped lettuce mixed with mayonnaise and vinegar.

For dessert: Add vanilla and sweetener to cream and whip until stiff. Alternate whipped cream in a parfait dish with layers of sliced raspberries or strawberries.

SHRIMP SCAMPI

Shrimp
Garlic salt
Butter
Spinach

Cream

Steam shrimp and weigh. Melt butter in dish with shrimp. Add pinch of garlic salt. Steam chopped spinach. Pat dry. Stir in some of cream if desired. Fix cream for beverage or dessert as desired.

CHICKEN SOUP AND CUSTARD

Diced chicken
Granulated bouillon
Carrots, celery, lettuce
Butter, mayonnaise
Egg
Cream
Salt (a speck)
Saccharin (1/8 grain)

Custard: Scald 3 parts cream to 1 part water. Combine with 2 parts beaten egg, salt, saccharin, and vanilla. Pour into a cup and bake in a shallow pan of water 25 minutes at 350° or until done (knife inserted in center will come out clean).

Soup: Dissolve bouillon cube in 1/2-cup hot water. Add enough chicken to make up the protein left over from the egg (if any) and carrots and celery to fill the carbohydrate allotment. Melt a little butter into the soup, and spread the rest of the fat as mayonnaise on lettuce. Drink any left-over cream as beverage.

IN THE CHICKEN SOUP RECIPE, the carrots can also be made into sticks and eaten dipped in mayonnaise instead of being diced into the soup.

CREAM OF TOMATO SOUP WITH GRILLED SWORDFISH

Tomato sauce
Cream
Speck of tarragon, salt, pepper
Lettuce leaf
Celery, onion
Fresh swordfish
Mayonnaise, Canola oil
Chocolate extract, sweetener

Sauté celery and onion in about 5 grams butter. Add tomato sauce. Add a speck each of tarragon, salt, and pepper. Add half of cream allotment and water to thin to desired consistency. Stir until smooth and heat until warm.

Meanwhile grill or broil seasoned swordfish, trim and weigh. Serve with a salad of chopped lettuce mixed with mayonnaise.

For dessert: Put chocolate extract drops into rest of cream and pour into bowl of ice cream scoop. Chill for 1 hour. Stir in canola oil quickly and return to freezer. Freeze until hard.

FOR A VARIETY OF CREAM SOUPS, Asparagus, broccoli, or spinach may be substituted for the tomato.

TREATS

BUTTER LOLLIPOPS

Soften butter. Add a tiny drop of vanilla and carbohydrate-free sweetener. Press into candy molds. Add lollipop sticks and freeze one hour or overnight. Calculate weight not including the sticks and serve with meals or snacks.

MACAROON COOKIES

2 Egg whites
1/2tsp. Cream of tartar
1/2 package Sugar-free Jell-O

Beat egg white until stiff. Add cream of tartar and dry Jell-O. Drop on aluminum foil sprayed lightly with nonstick cooking spray. Bake at 325° for 6 to 8 minutes, until brown. Cool before eating. Makes 20 cookies. One serving of two cookies contains 1.0g protein, 0g fat, and 0.1g carbohydrate.

MACADAMIA BUTTERCRUNCH

Chopped macadamia nuts
Butter

Macadamia nuts are naturally in a 3:1 ratio. Add enough butter to bring them to a 4:1 ratio. This snack is good for school kids and is easy to bring along on trips.

*EGGS BENEDICT**

[*Reproduced with permission from *The Ketogenic Cookbook* by Dennis and Cynthia Brake.]

Beaten egg
Grated cheddar cheese
Canadian bacon
Vanilla, sugar-free sweetener
Cream
Butter
Cantaloupe

Scramble eggs and weigh. Place on top of heated Canadian bacon. Top with butter and cheese. Melt in broiler or microwave. Serve with cantaloupe.

Frothy vanilla shake: In a blender, blend cream with a few drops of vanilla and sweetener and two ice cubes until ice is ground into a frothy shake.

"SPAGHETTI"

Spaghetti squash
Parmesan cheese
Lettuce
Hunt's tomato sauce
Ground beef or ground turkey
Butter
Mayonnaise
Cream
Zero-calorie flavored soda

Boil squash (raw squash may be frozen in individual portions in advance). Drain well and weigh. Cook and weigh ground meat, and sprinkle on squash. Melt butter with tomato sauce and some or all of cream. Pour on top. Sprinkle grated cheese plus a speck of pepper and oregano if desired. Mix chopped lettuce with mayonnaise for a salad.

Dessert: Pour any remaining cream in a zero-calorie flavored soda and whip lightly.

EVEN THE SMALLEST SPRINKLE of Parmesan cheese has to be calculated into the diet. Meatballs can be frozen for later use.

HOT DOG AND KETCHUP

Hebrew National hot dog
Zucchini or asparagus
Ketchup
Mayonnaise
Lettuce
Baking chocolate
Sugar-free Jell-O
Vanilla, sugar-free sweetener
Cream

Boil hot dog, drain, weigh. Mix ketchup with mayonnaise to make special sauce. Cut into thin slices; dab sauce on each slice. Arrange on a small plate. Steam vegetables; pat dry.

For dessert: (make in advance) Add a few drops of baking chocolate for flavoring, a little sweetener, and cream to the sugar-free Jell-O. Allow to set. Or make Keto Sherbet: Whip cream into sweetened Jell-O and freeze in the bowl of an ice cream scoop.

WITH COMMERCIAL PRODUCTS such as hot dogs, the brand must always be specified. Brands of hot dog other than Hebrew National may be used in this recipe if calculations are based on accurate information about the specified brand. Jell-O desserts are often calculated into hot dog meals to raise the protein.

BROILED STEAK WITH BROCCOLI

Steak
Broccoli
Butter
Mayonnaise
Cream
Orange flavored zero-calorie soda

Broil steak to medium rare. Weigh. Steam broccoli. Melt butter, blend with mayonnaise, pour over broccoli.

Serve with cream poured into orange flavored zero-calorie soda.

PEPPER STEAK STIR FRY AND BAVARIAN CREAM

Butter
Oil
Thin-sliced beef
Onions
Mushrooms
Green pepper
Speck of salt, pepper
Dash of soy sauce

Lettuce
Gelatin
Baking chocolate
Butter
Vanilla
Sugar-free sweetener

Bavarian cream: Swell 2 grams of gelatin with 2 tablespoons cold water. Add 2 grams baking chocolate and a little of allotted butter. Place over warm water until baking chocolate, butter, and gelatin are melted. Stir in 1/4 grain saccharin, a few drops vanilla, and cream. Pour into mold and freeze until hardened.

Stir fry: Heat oil equal to remaining fat allotment after butter used in Bavarian cream (some fat may be reserved for use as oil or mayonnaise in salad dressing). Sauté onions, mushrooms, and green pepper. Season with a speck of salt, pepper, and a dash of soy sauce. Cook beef separately in broiler or microwave. Weigh. Add to vegetables and serve. On the side, serve a chopped lettuce leaf with any remaining oil or mayonnaise for dressing.

IN THE BAVARIAN CREAM MEAL, total fat allotment is divided into three dishes. You can decide how much butter to melt into the Bavarian cream, how much oil to use with the stir-fry, and how much oil or mayonnaise to use as salad dressing as long as all fats add up to the correct total.

BURGER WITH "POTATO SALAD"

Ground beef
Zucchini
Ketchup
Mayonnaise, oil
Salt, pepper
Oregano
Lettuce
Vanilla, sweetener
Sugar-free Jell-O

Flatten the ground beef into a 1/4-inch thick burger. Heat a nonstick skillet with a few drops of the allotted oil or cooking spray. Sauté the burger 1 to 1–1/2 minutes on each side. Weigh the sautéed burger and trim. Meanwhile, measure the ketchup and beat in an equal amount of oil. Steam zucchini. Weigh and cut into 1/2-inch cubes. Mix the zucchini with mayonnaise, oregano, and a pinch of salt and pepper. Arrange the beef on a lettuce leaf. Spread ketchup mixture on steak.

For Dessert: Top sugar-free Jell-O with whipped sweetened vanilla cream.

I BOUGHT THE KIND OF BLENDER that's a wand you can stick right into a tall glass. You just rinse the wand off in the sink after you use it. That way I don't have to wash the whole blender every time.

"PIZZA"

Egg
Tomato puree
Lettuce
Olive oil
Mozzarella cheese
Pepperoni or ground beef
Speck of oregano
Cream
Vanilla, sweetener

Beat egg with cream. Pour into heated non-stick pan. Spread thinly. Turn heat to low and let sit until hardened. Mix olive oil with tomato sauce; spread on egg crust. Sprinkle with a speck of oregano. Cover with grated cheese. Top with pepperoni or ground beef. Broil until melted.

Serve with diluted cream shake. Note: A thin slice of eggplant, broiled, can serve as crust for alternative recipe.

A THIN TOMATO SLICE may be substituted for the egg-cream or eggplant pizza crust. Triangular slices of cheese can also make a fun pretend pizza!

BROILED FISH WITH TARTAR SAUCE

Flounder or other fish
Lettuce
Tartar sauce
Butternut squash
Butter, mayonnaise
Accent, pepper
Sugar-free Jell-O
Cream

Broil the fish about 5 minutes or until flaky. Season with a speck of Accent and pepper. Spread with measured tartar sauce. Bake butternut squash or cook frozen puree. Melt butter into squash puree. Arrange flounder on a small plate with squash and chopped lettuce with mayonnaise.

Dessert: Serve sugar-free Jell-O topped with whipped cream.

I DON'T COOK WITH BUTTER as the allowed fat. Because the fat is his body fuel, I want him to get as much as possible. When you cook with butter, you can easily lose some of it in the pan. I usually just spray the pan with nonstick aerosol spray, cook the food, and add the butter while it's hot.

CHICKEN FINGERS AND COLE SLAW

Oil

Chicken breast
Butter
Dash of mustard, tarragon, and garlic salt
Cabbage
Carrot
Scallion
Lettuce
Mayonnaise
Vinegar
Cream
Vanilla, sweetener

Heat a few drops oil in a nonstick skillet. Sauté chicken breast at medium-high heat for about 3 minutes per side or until lightly browned. Remove chicken from heat; weigh and trim. Turn heat off. Add butter (1/3 of fat allotment) to skillet. Add a dash of mustard, tarragon, and garlic salt. Stir until butter is melted. Remove skillet from heat. Cut chicken breast into thin strips or very thin slices and fan out on a small plate. Pour butter sauce over chicken. Meanwhile, chop cabbage (red or green) with a little grated carrot, thinly sliced scallion, and a leaf of lettuce. Mix mayonnaise (2/3 of fat allotment) with a couple of grams of vinegar. Stir in cabbage mixture. Sprinkle with salt and pepper.

For Dessert: Serve with frozen vanilla-flavored cream ball.

BEEF STEW

Roast beef
Pearl onions
Cabbage
Cherry tomatoes
Turnips
Cream
Baking chocolate
Sugar-free sweetener

Steam cabbage, turnip, and onion until tender. Place them in a small, nonstick pot (such as a one-cup Pyrex) with the roast beef and 1/4 cup water. Add butter and sprinkle with a speck of salt and pepper. Simmer 15 minutes. For thicker sauce, mash some turnip into the liquid. Place cherry tomato halves around a small plate and spoon stew in center.

For Dessert: Serve with chocolate ice cream made from baking chocolate, cream, and sweetener.

CHICKEN CUTLET WITH APPLE À LA MODE

Chicken
Butter/Mayonnaise
Lettuce
Apple slice

Cream
Cinnamon
Saccharin

Chicken cutlet: Pound the chicken very thin between sheets of waxed paper. Grill or pan fry for 1 minute on each side. Sprinkle with a speck of seasoned salt or salt and pepper, and dot with some of allotted butter if desired. Spread lettuce leaf with butter or mayonnaise, roll into a pinwheel, cut in half, and arrange on small plate with chicken.

Apple à la mode: Cut center slice from a small apple. Leave skin on, remove core, and weigh. Sauté in remaining butter in a small skillet until soft. Dust with a speck of cinnamon. Place apple slice in an ice cream dish and top with a ball of sweetened vanilla frozen cream made from cream and saccharin. Pour any cinnamon butter remaining in skillet on top of ice cream. *(Optional:* Serve with Shasta red apple diet drink.)

CHICKEN WITH MASHED TURNIPS

Chicken breast
Vegetable oil
Turnips
Butter
Salt, pepper
Tarragon or oregano (optional)
Leaf lettuce

Cream

Broil chicken breast or sauté it in a nonstick skillet with a few drops of oil. Season chicken with a few flakes of tarragon or oregano if desired. Boil turnips until soft. Mash with butter. Season with salt and pepper. Serve with a chopped lettuce leaf and diluted cream.

CHRIS LOVED MASHED BUTTERED TURNIPS because they reminded him of potatoes, and he loved potatoes even though he couldn't have them.

LAMB WITH CUCUMBER AND TOMATO SALAD

Lamb chop
Pepper
Accent
Rosemary (optional)
Cucumber
Tomato
Vinegar
Olive oil
Leaf lettuce
Mayonnaise

Broil lamb chop 4 minutes on each side. Season with a speck of pepper and Accent or rosemary if desired. Trim off fat and weigh lamb. Slice meat thinly and fan out on plate. Cut cucumber and tomato into 1/2-inch cubes. Combine vinegar and olive oil and pour over cucumber-tomato salad. Serve on a chopped or rolled lettuce leaf spread with mayonnaise.

"TACOS"

Ground beef
Speck of chili powder
Lettuce
Cream
Orange diet soda
Chopped tomato
Grated cheese or sour cream

Cook beef in nonstick pan. Weigh. Dust beef with a speck of chili powder. Roll beef, tomato, and cheese or sour cream in lettuce leaf.

Dessert drink: Pour cream into up to 120 grams of orange diet soda.

EVERY WEEKEND I WOULD MAKE 21 ICE CREAM SERVINGS. My son didn't like much fat in his meals, so I hid almost all of it in the ice cream, which he loved and ate with every meal. I had to plan my menus in advance so I would know how much fat I had to hide in the ice cream for each meal. Mostly I used canola oil, which whips into the cream beautifully just before it freezes. There would be different quantities of oil whipped in with the cream, depending on each menu. Sometimes I would choose a menu with fruit and make strawberry ice cream. I had to label the ice cream very carefully as to which day and which meal they were made for.

KETO WAFFLE WITH "SYRUP"

Egg yolk
Egg white
Cream
Sweetener
Nonstick vegetable oil spray
Butter
Carbohydrate-free pure Maple flavoring

Mix egg yolk, whipped egg whites, and whipped cream together with a few drops of sweetener. Pour into the center of a heated waffle iron sprayed with nonstick cooking spray. Melt butter with maple flavoring for syrup.

KETO DONUT

Egg whites
Macadamia nuts, finely chopped
Peanut butter
Cream, whipped
Butter

Spray mini bundt pans with nonstick cooking spray. Mix egg whites, whipped cream and nuts, set aside. Melt butter and peanut butter together—mix well—and pour into the egg mixture. Pour into mini bundt pans and bake at 350° for about 30 minutes.

JELL-O MOLD

Sugar-free Jell-O
Cream
Cream cheese
Sour cream
Butter
1/4g Saccharin (optional)

Make Jell-O ahead of time and start to cool in the refrigerator. Meanwhile, whip cream. Whip in softened cream cheese, sour cream, and butter. Add 1/4 gram saccharin if desired. Stir into cool liquid Jell-O and let harden. Note: This menu is helpful for children who do not chew well. Every bite is ketogenic, which means it can also be used for children during illness.

BECAUSE CREAM contains so much fat, the more cream you use the less oil, mayonnaise, and butter you will have to fit into the rest of the menu. But if your child doesn't mind eating a lot of mayonnaise or butter, you can use less cream and fill out the carbohydrate allotment with more vegetables or fruit.

CHEESECAKE: A BIRTHDAY MEAL!

Egg
Cottage cheese
Sour cream
Cream cheese
Butter
Cream
Vanilla Sweetener
Fruit slices

Mix together all ingredients except fruit. Add vanilla to taste and 1/2 grain of saccharin dissolved in 1/2 teaspoon of warm water or liquid sweetener to taste. Bake in small, greased Pyrex dish at 350° for 25 minutes or until light golden on top. Cool. Arrange fruit slices on top—sliced strawberries, pineapple, or peach. Makes a whole meal! Save a bit of cream to whip and pile on top for extra excitement.

A CHEESECAKE MEAL is easy to carry to school in its container for special occasions, such as when other kids are eating cake to celebrate a birthday. Cheesecake also provides a ketogenic ratio in every bite, so it is useful for children who cannot eat a full meal (e.g., when recovering from an illness).

THANKSGIVING CUSTARD

Turkey breast
Turnip*
Butter
Green beans*
Egg
Cream
Canned pumpkin
Dash of cinnamon
Sugar-free sweetener

Weigh cooked turkey breast. Mash turnip with butter. Top green beans and/or turkey with rest of butter.

Dessert: Whip egg, cream, canned pumpkin, dash of cinnamon, and sweetener. Bake at 325° in Pyrex dish. *Note: Cranberry sauce may be calculated into the menu, replacing both green beans and turnip.

KETOGENIC EGGNOG

Cream
Vanilla
Egg
Saccharin

Beat egg slightly. Weigh. Dissolve saccharin in 1 teaspoon or more water. Add to cream. Combine egg, cream, vanilla, and sweetener to taste. Whip lightly if desired. Sprinkle with nutmeg. Use as travel meal or for an occasional snack. When put in the microwave, eggnog turns into a loose scrambled egg consistency.

LIKE THE CHEESECAKE, frozen eggnog in a margarine tub makes a great birthday party food. Try decorating top with fruit (strawberries, cherries). Wrap the margarine tub in colored foil and take it to school for birthday parties.

SNACKS

PEANUT BUTTER BALLS

Skippy creamy peanut butter
Butter

Mix peanut butter and butter together. Roll out into little balls and place in the fridge for a quick snack.

KETO YOGURT

Cream
Fruit
Sugar-free sweetener (optional)
Sour cream

Mix all of the ingredients together in the blender. Or mix the cream and sour cream together and place chopped up fruit in the mixture. You can add a sweetener as well.

JELL-O AND WHIPPED CREAM

Cream (whipped)
Sugar-free Jell-O

Mix or whip together, you can place it in the freezer for a frozen snack.

CUSTARD (BAKED OR FROZEN) OR EGGNOG SNACK

Eggs Whole (raw)
Cream
Saccharin drops to sweeten
Pure extract: vanilla, almond, or chocolate, etc.

Whip the eggs, add the rest of the ingredients, and bake.

TURKEY OR HAM ROLLUP

Turkey breast or ham
Mayonnaise
Iceberg lettuce
Avocado (optional)

Spread mayonnaise on a lettuce leaf and roll turkey or ham in it. For variations you can add avocado into the wrap.

CHOCOLATE BAVARIAN

Cream (whipped)
Unsweetened cocoa powder
Knox unflavored gelatin
Saccharin drops to sweeten
Pure chocolate extract

Swell gelatin in cold water. Add saccharin, whipped cream, and chocolate extract. Pour into a ramekin or mold and refrigerate until Bavarian sets.

PEANUT BUTTER MUFFINS WITH KETO ICING

Egg yolk
Egg white
Pam nonstick vegetable oil spray
Butter
Skippy creamy peanut butter
Vanilla extract
Saccharin drops to sweeten

*Recipe makes **3** servings

Spray a miniature muffin/tart pan with Pam nonstick vegetable oil. Separate the yolk from the white of the egg. Whip the egg white until it is fluffy and measure allotted amount. Fold in allotted egg yolk. Melt butter with the peanut butter. Blend the melted butter and peanut butter with the egg mixture. Spoon it into the pan to make 9 little mini muffins. Bake at 350 for 10–15 minutes. Take them out and let them stand until the butter gets absorbed into the muffins. One serving equals 3 muffins

Keto-Icing: For a variation you could try setting a little butter from the recipe aside, mix it with vanilla extract and a few drops of saccharin, and spread it on top of the muffins.

QUESTIONS ABOUT PREPARING THE DIET

Q: *Is it good to use high-fat meats to increase the fat content of the diet?*

A: Protein is very important for your child's growth. The protein portion of the diet should therefore be close to pure. Meat should be lean and trimmed of fat. Chicken and fish should be without skin. Cooked fat may be trimmed off and measured separately as part of the fat allotment for the meal. High-fat processed meats such as sausage and bologna should be calculated in the menu according to the manufacturer's contents.

Q: *What if some of the food sticks to the pan?*

A: Use nonstick pans and nonstick spray, and scrape out as much as possible with a small rubber spatula. Cook at low temperatures to avoid burning. Better yet, prepare food using nonstick methods: bake or broil meats, microwave eggs, steam vegetables. Remember that the allotted weights are for cooked food unless otherwise indicated, so until you are experienced with the difference between raw and cooked weights, your meats and vegetables or fruits should be prepared and cooked separately and then assembled with fats at the end.

Q: *What if my child refuses to eat the food I make?*

A: It is almost unheard of for a child to go hungry on the ketogenic diet. Remember that you are in charge, not the child! If your child has a tantrum and refuses to eat the food, give it 20–30 minutes, then remove the meal and you finish the family meal. Odds are, by the next meal, your child will not be so willing to test your limits and will eat the food.

If meal battles persist, allow the child some say in choosing the food (e.g., popular choices such as hot dogs, tuna fish, etc.). Another great trick (used by pediatricians for years!) is to have your child help in the actual meal preparation (e.g., mixing mayonnaise in with tuna, counting out pieces of vegetables). Try to make the child an actual participant in the diet, not just a recipient!

Q: *Should I try to use margarine instead of butter?*

A: We recommend that you use as many unsaturated fats as possible, such as canola, safflower, flaxseed, or olive oil, or margarine made from canola oil. However, no research exists on the effect of a diet comprised of 90% fat, whether saturated or unsaturated. No data indicate that the ketogenic diet, despite its high fat content, leads to heart disease or atherosclerosis later in life.

Q: *My child is too disabled to care much what she eats, so I just want the simplest menu to prepare. What is easiest?*

A: The simplest ketogenic menu planning involves using the four main food groups of the diet without embellishment:

- Protein (meat, fish, chicken, cheese, egg)
- Carbohydrate (fruit or vegetable)
- Fat (butter, margarine, mayonnaise, oil)
- Cream

It takes very little time to broil a bit of meat or chicken, steam a piece of broccoli or cut up a tomato, put butter on the chicken or mayonnaise on the broccoli, and serve with a cup of cream diluted with ice and water. For a softer consistency, try fruit-topped cheesecake or custard with bacon and cooked vegetables.

Q: *What if the family has to travel or I don't have time to prepare a meal?*

A: The eggnog recipe or Ketocal® recipe that you receive from your dietitian is a very good emergency or convenience food on the ketogenic diet. Chopped macadamia nuts mixed with butter can also be eaten for an occasional meal. You should not use these meals too often in the diet, but they can tide you over in a pinch. When traveling, take up to 2 days' meals ahead of time and take them along in a portable cooler. Ask restaurants to microwave them for you if appropriate. Tuna salad with sliced vegetables such as celery, cucumbers, or carrots is especially mobile. See Chapter 6 for further details.

Q: *Can I decrease the amount of cream and use more fat in a given menu?*

A: Cream is an easy, palatable way to get a lot of fat into the diet. If desired, however, the diet can be calculated with little or no cream. The challenge will be to find ways to make a large quantity of fats or oils palatable.

Q: *My child only wants to eat bacon and hot dogs, is that OK?*

A: As long as she is taking her vitamins and minerals it is ok for her to eat the same foods every day. There are no set meals for breakfast or dinner; each meal plan is interchangeable and can be eaten for any meal.

Q: *What if my child only ate the strawberries and then refused to eat the rest of the meal?*

A: Your child could be refusing to eat for many reasons. If it's out of pure control and refusal, then follow the guidelines above and discard the meal. However, in the future you should try and give the fats first and then save the fruit as a dessert for the end of the meal, this way you don't have to worry about fighting with your child to get the required fat in. Some meals have all the ingredients mixed in together, and if your child might not finish a complete meal at times, it might be best to prepare those meals for her. This way you know that she had the entire ratio but just didn't finish all of her calories for that meal.

CHAPTER TWENTY THREE

Modified Atkins Diet Recipes

These recipes are donated courtesy of many families that have found them helpful for their child's time on the Atkins diet. Some of these can be found on the Web site www.atkinsforseizures.com. Thanks to Michael Koski for allowing us to use these. Others near the end are from Nutricia North America's KetoCal® Web site, www.myketocal.com, with the help of Chef Neil Palliser-Bosomworth.

For other great recipes ideas, go to the Atkins approach Web site, www.atkins.com. Also, read Chapter 22, and use the recipes listed there for children on the ketogenic diet (just don't worry about portions and calories and only keep the proportions of food amounts the same). Happy eating!

CHOCOLATE MACADAMIA NUT MUFFINS (LOOK JUST LIKE CHOCOLATE CUPCAKES)

6 egg whites
6 egg yolks
1/2tsp cream of tartar
Liquid Sweet & Low® 70 drops—divided

1/4 cup Carbsense zero carb baking mix™ (or other low carb
baking mix—soy flour will work)
2tsp cocoa—sifted
1/4 cup macadamia nuts—finely chopped
1tsp vanilla

Frosting

4oz cream cheese
3tbsp cream—or less
3tbsp Keto hot cocoa mix
1tsp vanilla
1/4 cup macadamia nuts—finely chopped

Separate the eggs and put the whites into mixer bowl. Add the cream of tartar and 35 drops of Sweet & Low; beat until stiff peaks form. In a separate bowl mix the egg and vanilla and beat well. Stir together the flour, cocoa, nuts, and remaining Sweet & Low; add to the egg yolks and stir well. Add a good-sized spoonful of the whites to the yolks to thin the batter down. Carefully fold the batter into the egg whites, being careful not to deflate the whites.

Spray 12 muffin tins with nonstick spray, then carefully spoon the batter into them; do not flatten. Bake in a pre-heated 350°F–180°C oven for 25 minutes. Remove from oven and cool on a wire rack. When cool, beat the frosting together till creamy. Spread frosting on muffins and sprinkle the nuts over top.

FRENCH TOAST

1/2 of a 3-oz bag of unflavored pork rinds
2 eggs
1/4 cup heavy cream
3 packets sweetener
1/2tsp cinnamon
1/2tsp egg nog extract (optional)

Crumble pork rinds up until they resemble bread crumbs (use your food processor or put them in a Ziploc bag—air removed—and roll them with a rolling pin.) Set aside.

Beat eggs well and then mix with remaining ingredients and beat again. Add crushed pork rinds to the egg/cream mixture and allow to sit for approximately 5 minutes. Mixture will thicken.

Meanwhile, heat skillet or griddle with butter or oil, and when hot, fry pancake style until golden brown on both sides. Serve with your favorite zero-carb maple syrup.

Notes: For the best flavor, use pork rinds with a bland taste. It's also important that you crush them well—until they are almost the texture of dust. Lastly, the egg nog extract is optional, but does add a nice flavor. If you don't have any, use vanilla. Recipe makes two servings.

CHEESEBURGER PIE

1lb ground beef, scant onion powder
1tbs heavy whipping cream (add enough water to make 1 1/2 cups liquid)
3/4 cup Carbsense zero carb baking mix™
3 medium eggs
1/2tsp salt
1/4tsp pepper
1 cup shredded cheese
1tbs prepared yellow mustard (optional)

In a 10″ iron skillet, cook the hamburger and onion powder over medium heat. Break the meat up into smallish pieces with a fork, and cook it until there is no more pink showing. Drain off the fat if necessary. While the meat is cooking get out a medium-sized bowl. In it combine the milk, baking mix, eggs, salt, and pepper. Mix very well with a whisk, or combine it in a blender. You want it pretty smooth. When the meat is well cooked and drained, put into prepared pie plate. You can put mustard on top if you'd like, pour the batter over it. Sprinkle the cheese on top. Bake the dish at 400° for about 35 minutes, longer if need be. It should be puffed up and brown on top when it is done.

Remove the pan from the oven and cut it into 8 wedges.

DEEP DISH PIZZA

4oz cream cheese, softened
2 eggs
1/4 cup parmesan cheese, 1 ounce (I used the kind in a can)
1/4tsp oregano or Italian seasoning
1/4tsp garlic powder
8ozs Italian cheese blend or mozzarella cheese, shredded
1/4 cup pizza sauce
4ozs mozzarella cheese, shredded
Assorted toppings: pepperoni, ham, sausage, 4oz can mushrooms, green peppers, bacon, ground beef, etc.
Dash of garlic powder and some Italian seasoning for top of pizza

In a medium bowl, whisk cream cheese until smooth and creamy. Whisk in eggs until mixture is well-blended and smooth. Add the parmesan and seasonings, then stir in the 8 ounces of mozzarella until completely moistened. Spread cheese mixture evenly in a well-greased 9x13" glass baking dish. Bake at 375° for 20–25 minutes or until evenly browned, but not too dark. Let cool completely on a wire rack. When nearly cooled, take a metal spatula and carefully pry up the edges to loosen from pan. Ease the spatula under the whole crust to loosen. Keep crust in the pan. This makes it easier to remove the finished pizza later. Refrigerate, uncovered, until shortly before serving time. Spread chilled crust with pizza sauce, then cheese and toppings of your choice. Lightly sprinkle with seasonings of your choice. Bake at 375 about 15–20 minutes or until toppings are bubbly. Let stand a few minutes before cutting.

FAUX FRIED RICE

Fresh head of cauliflower
1 egg
Olive oil
3 to 4 scallions
ZERO carb soy sauce

Grate one head of fresh cauliflower (or a bag of frozen and put through a food processor)—*do not use cooked cauliflower* as it gets too mushy. Sauté 3–4 green scallions in olive oil. Add the grated cauliflower. Sauté till the veggies are tender, then add a few tablespoons of ZERO-carb soy sauce (carefully check the label as brands vary widely). Beat one egg and blend it into the mixture. Stir until the egg is cooked and blended into the mixture. Serve.

LEMON CAPER SALAD DRESSING

3tbsp freshly squeezed lemon juice
1 clove garlic, minced
2tbsp capers, finely chopped
1tbsp caper juice from jar
1/2 cup good fruity olive oil

Place garlic into processor bowl. Mince. Add capers. Mince. Add lemon juice and caper juice. Process. With processor running, add oil slowly through feed tube, blending well. This keeps well in a jar in the refrigerator for at least 2 weeks.

TURNIP FRIES

Slice and peel 8 turnips as you would potatoes for fries. Place the turnips in a bowl and pour 1/2 cup of heavy cream over them. Add 10–20 drops of liquid Sweet & Low and enough cold water to cover the turnips. Let them soak for 1/2 hour, then drain, rinse, and pat dry (this process will eliminate their bitter taste). Spray a large cookie sheet heavily with baking spray. Put the following seasonings into a large plastic zip lock bag: 1/4 cup Parmesan cheese, 1tsp. Mrs. Dash seasoning (Or Adobo w/Pepper or Kosher Salt) 1/4tsp grated nutmeg and pepper. Shake the turnips in the bag to coat them. Spread them on the baking sheet and drizzle them with olive oil or spray them with cooking spray. Bake them in a hot 425° oven for

15 minutes. Turn them and bake another 15 minutes. Give them a quick squirt with a slice of fresh lime before serving.

FAUX MAC AND CHEESE

1 bag frozen cauliflower, cooked
3ozs cream cheese
2tsps heavy cream
1 cup shredded cheddar

Preheat oven to 350°. Pour a little cream in bottom of baking dish and add a handful of cheddar cheese. Place cream, cream cheese, and remaining cheese in microwave safe dish and microwave, stirring every 30 seconds or so, until all can be stirred together easily. Pour drained cauliflower into baking dish (while cauliflower is still hot). Pour cheese mixture over and stir well to mix. Sprinkle some parmesan over top. Bake 35 minutes; allow to stand few minutes before eating/serving. Recipe makes two servings as a main dish; four as a side dish.

CARB-FRIENDLY GREEK SALAD

Romaine lettuce
Olive oil
1/4tsp red wine vinegar
Feta cheese
Sliced olives

2–3 sliced cucumbers

PEANUT BUTTER COOKIES

1/2 cup (plus) natural creamy peanut butter
1/4 cup room temp butter
2 eggs
2/3 cup heavy whipping cream
1/2tsp baking soda
1/4tsp sea salt
Stevia to taste (We use about 20 drops)

Bake at 375° for 11 minutes. (May be a bit different for the lowlanders.)

CHOCOLATE ICE CREAM

38gm 36% heaving whipping cream (whipped)
2gm hershey's unsweetened cocoa powder
1gm canola oil
1gm unflavored Knox gelatin

BROWNIES

4ozs unsweetened chocolate (can be any brand Hersheys, etc., as long as unsweetened)
1 1/2 sticks of butter
Bickford's vanilla flavoring—about 1 1/2tsps
1 cup Splenda or NoSugar
1 cup of almond flour

3 eggs

Melt chocolate and butter together in microwave or over a pan with boiling water. Blend well. Add sugar and vanilla until well blended.

Last step is to blend in eggs, then almond flour. Bake in well-greased 8x8x2 baking pan at 350° for 30–35 minutes or until toothpick comes out almost clean.

SHRIMP SCAMPI

Shelled shrimp
1/4 stick of butter
1tsp chopped garlic
1/4tsp cilantro
1/4 cup dry white wine
1/2tsp lemon juice
1tsp olive oil
Salt and pepper

Heat butter and oil over low heat, add shrimp and cook until pink. Add garlic for 1 additional minute. Then add wine, lemon juice, salt, and pepper.

ASPARAGUS, LIMA BEAN, AND SALAMI SALAD

(FROM ATKINS.COM)
8 servings, 4.5 grams of carbohydrates/serving

2 bunches asparagus (30 spears), trimmed and steamed (about 2lb)
2tbsp extra-virgin olive oil
1tsp chopped garlic
1tsp fresh rosemary, finely chopped
1tsp freshly grated lemon zest (1 lemon)
3/4tsp salt
1/2tsp freshly ground black pepper
1 cup frozen baby lima beans, cooked
2ozs Genoa salami, cut into matchstick pieces (about 2/3 cup)

Directions

1. In lightly salted boiling water, cook asparagus 3 to 5 minutes, until tender-crisp. Drain into a colander and shock under cold running water for 3 minutes. Allow excess water to drain, stack in bundles and cut into 1″ pieces. Place in a large bowl.
2. In the same bowl, add oil, garlic, rosemary, lemon zest, salt, and pepper. Add lima beans and salami; toss to coat.

MINI MEXICAN PIZZA SQUARES

(FROM ATKINS.COM)

10 servings, 4 grams of carbohydrates/serving
10 slices Atkins bakery country white bread™
1 1/2tsp olive oil

1 cup shredded monterey jack cheese
1/2 cup tomato salsa
2 green onions, very thinly sliced
6 black pitted black olives, sliced
2tbsp chopped fresh cilantro

Directions

1. Heat oven to 400° F. Trim crusts from bread (save to make bread crumbs). Brush bread with olive oil on one side and lightly toast.
2. Cut each slice into four pieces. Arrange squares on a baking sheet. Divide cheese on toast squares; top cheese with a scant tablespoon of salsa. Sprinkle with green onions and olives.
3. Bake 10 minutes until cheese is bubbly. Sprinkle cilantro over pizzas squares. Serve immediately.

RASPBERRY CHEESECAKE IN A CUP

(FROM ATKINS.COM)

4 servings, 5 grams of carbohydrates/serving

Cheesecakes

1 package (8ozs) cream cheese, at room temperature
2 large eggs
1/2 cup heavy cream
3 packets Splenda™
1/4tsp almond extract

1/4tsp freshly grated lemon peel

Topping

1/2 pint fresh raspberries
3tbsp Atkins sugar free raspberry syrup™

Directions

1. Heat oven to 325°F. Place four 6-ounce custard cups in a large roasting pan.
2. Process all cheesecake ingredients in a food processor until smooth, stopping when necessary to scrape down sides of processor.
3. Pour batter into cups. Add enough boiling water to roasting pan to come halfway up sides of cups. Cover with foil; bake 30 minutes. Turn oven off and let stand 20 minutes. Remove from oven, uncover and cool completely. Cover cups with plastic wrap; transfer to refrigerator to chill.
4. When ready to serve, toss raspberries with syrup. Evenly top cheesecakes with raspberries. Let stand at room temperature 15 minutes before serving for maximum creaminess.

CREAMY CRAB DIP (A BALTIMORE FAVORITE!)

(FROM ATKINS.COM)

6 servings, 1 gram of carbohydrate/serving

1/4 cup mayonnaise
1/4 cup full-fat sour cream
1tsp old bay seasoning
1tsp fresh lemon juice
1 can (6ozs) white crab meat, drained and picked over
2 green onions, finely chopped
2tbsp chopped red bell pepper
Salt
Freshly ground pepper

Directions

In a medium bowl, mix mayonnaise, sour cream, seasoning, and lemon juice until smooth. Add crab, green onions, and pepper; stir until ingredients are well combined. Season to taste with salt and pepper.

These recipes are from myketocal.com/recipes_mad.html

CHEESE PIZZA, MODIFIED ATKINS DIET (MADE WITH KETOCAL® 3:1)

Kcal	CHO	Fat	Pro	Ratio
286	2.89	28.08	5.25	3.45.1

Ingredient List (includes pizza crust and topping combined)

1/4 cup	Ketocal® 3:1 powder—Nutricia North America
1tbsp	egg—raw—mixed well
1tbsp	olive oil
2tsp	water
1/2tsp	garlic paste—Amore®
1/2tsp	tomato paste—sun-dried—Amore®
1tbsp	tomatoes—canned, diced, undrained
1/2tbsp	hard parmesan cheese, grated pinch of dried italian herbs (optional)

Pizza Crust

1/4 cup	Ketocal® 3:1 powder—Nutricia North America
1tbsp	egg—raw—mixed well
1tbsp	olive oil

2tsp	water

Instructions for Pizza Crust

- Preheat oven to 325°F.
- In a small bowl, combine and mix all the ingredients together.
- Spread the mixture onto a lightly greased baking sheet in a 5-inch circle and set aside.

Pizza Topping

1/2tsp	garlic paste—Amore®
1/2tsp	tomato paste—sun-dried—Amore®
1tbsp	tomatoes—canned, diced, undrained
1/2tbsp	hard parmesan cheese, grated pinch of dried italian herbs (optional)

Instructions for Pizza Toppings

- In a bowl, combine and mix the garlic paste, tomato paste, and tomatoes together.
- Spread the mixture on top of the pizza crust evenly, leaving a 1/2-inch space around the edge free of toppings.
- Sprinkle all of the grated parmesan cheese and a pinch of dried Italian herbs on the top of the pizza.

- Bake for about 10 to 12 minutes.

MUSHROOM AND SPINACH CURRY, MODIFIED ATKINS DIET (MADE WITH KETOCAL® 3:1)

Kcal	CH	Fat	Pro	Ratio
284	4.45	27.21	5.48	2.74:1

1/2tsp	garlic paste—Amore®
1/4 cup	mushrooms, white—raw—finely chopped
1tbsp	olive oil
2tbsp	peppers, green—raw, chopped
1/4 cup	onions, spring or scallions (tops only)—raw, chopped
1/2tsp	tomato paste—sun-dried—Amore®
1/2tsp	curry powder
2tbsp	tomatoes—canned, diced, undrained
1 cup	spinach leaf—raw
1tbsp	water
1/4 cup	Ketocal® 3:1 powder—Nutricia North America

Instructions

- Heat olive oil in a pan over medium-low heat. Add the mushrooms, peppers, spring onions, tomato paste, and garlic paste, and cook for 5 minutes on medium heat or until soft.

• Add the chopped tomatoes, curry powder, spinach, and water. Cook for 5 minutes on low heat stirring frequently.

• Add KetoCal® into curry and mix vigorously with a utensil until smooth. Do not boil when KetoCal® is in curry.

Chef's Tip

Add Curry powder to the KetoCal® Tomato Wrap, put the curry in the middle, fold, and enjoy!

Makes 1 serving.

BLUEBERRY MUFFINS, MODIFIED ATKINS DIET (MADE WITH KETOCAL® 4:1)

(Recipe adapted from Emma Williams' recipe collection from Matthews Friends)

Per Serving (1 muffin)

Kcal	CHO	Fat	Pro	Ratio
190	1.66	18.64	3.77	3.43:1

Recipe (3 muffins)

Kcal	CHO	Fat	Pro	Ratio
569	4.98	55.92	11.32	3.43:1

3 1/2tbsp	cream, 36%—heavy whipping cream
1 1/2tbsp	blueberries, fresh
2 1/2tbsp	egg—raw—mixed well
1/3 cup	Ketocal® 4:1 powder—Nutricia North America
3tbsp	almond fl our (whole ground blanched almonds)*
2tbsp	butter
1tbsp	water
3 drops	liquid sweetener

Instructions

- Preheat oven to 325°F.
- Mix together the dry ingredients: KetoCal® powder and almond flour.*
- In a separate container, melt the butter. Allow to cool for approximately 1 minute.
- Mix egg, cream, and water into melted butter until well blended.
- Stir mixture into dry ingredients.
- If desired, stir in several drops of liquid sweetener.**
- Fold in blueberries
- Spoon mixture into foil muffin cups in a muffin tin.
- Bake for 20 minutes.
- Refrigerate in a sealed bag for up to 2 days. Muffin may be frozen.

*Almond flour is the same as almond meal; whole ground blanched almonds.

**Liquid sweeteners such as Sweet 10®, Sweet'n Low®, or Stevia®.

RASPBERRY CRUMBLE, MODIFIED ATKINS DIET (MADE WITH KETOCAL® 4:1)

Kcal	CHO	Fat	Pro	Ratio
358	3.83	35.98	4.76	4.19:1

1/2 cup	raspberries
1tbsp	butter
1/4 cup	Ketocal® 4:1 powder—nutricia north america
1/4 cup	coconut—dried, shredded—unsweetened
	Carbohydrate-free sweetener (optional)
	Pinch of cinnamon (optional)

Instructions

- Preheat oven to 300°F.
- Mix softened butter, KetoCal®, and coconut together with your fingertips. The mixture should look like fine breadcrumbs.
- If desired, add in carbohydrate-free sweetener and/or a pinch of cinnamon to above mixture.
- Place the raw raspberries in a small, oven proof ramekin.

- Spread crumble on top of raspberries in ramekin.
- Bake in preheated oven for 15-20 minutes or until golden brown.

Makes 1 serving.

PANCAKES OR WAFFLES, MODIFIED ATKINS DIET (MADE WITH KETOCAL® 4:1)

(Recipe adapted from Emma Williams' recipe collection from Matthews Friends)

Per Serving (1 Pancake or Waffle):

Kcal	CHO	Fat	Pro	Ratio
126	1.32	12.24	2.64	3.09:1

Recipe (3 Pancakes or Waffles, 4" diameter):

Kcal	CHO	Fat	Pro	Ratio
378	3.96	36.72	7.93	3.09:1

3tbsp	cream, 36%—heavy whipping cream
3tbsp	blueberries, fresh
1tbsp	egg yolk—raw—mixed well
2 1/2tbsp	egg white—raw*—whipped
3tsp	butter
1/4 cup	ketocal® 4:1—nutricia north america

1tbsp	water

*1 large egg contains approximately 1/4 cup of egg white. When egg white is whipped, it will expand several times in volume.

Instructions

- Melt butter; stir in egg yolk, cream, and water until well blended.
- Mix KetoCal® powder into above mixture.
- Whip the egg white from 1 large egg and then weigh out 1tbsp+2tsp.
- Fold egg white into batter.
- Fold in blueberries.
- Spray small frying pan or waffle iron with oil spray and warm to medium heat. Fry batter to desired doneness.
- Very tasty if served with melted butter flavored with several drops of carbohydrate free maple flavoring such as Bickford.

SECTION VI

The Future of Diets and the Brain

CHAPTER TWENTY FOUR

Can the Diet Be Used Before Medications?

Despite its proven efficacy in the treatment of so-called intractable childhood epilepsy (seizure disorders that have failed to respond to the proper use of three or more anticonvulsant medications), the ketogenic diet is still regarded as the "treatment of last resort" by many neurologists and other physicians who manage seizure patients. As the diet gains more popularity around the world, studies have shown that some of the old myths about how the diet can be used are incorrect.

We now know that the ketogenic diet can be helpful in the treatment of both generalized and partial seizures, although it is less likely to be as completely effective in the localization-related (partial) epilepsies. It can be successfully implemented in a wide range of ages without any clear influence of age on outcome. There is value in using dietary therapy short term in children who may ultimately require surgical intervention, especially when they are young children. It may have value in such cases for status epilepticus, in fact.

The ketogenic diet can be used as "first-line" therapy in certain situations, and actually there is agreement that it is the "treatment of choice" in specific epilepsy syndromes. The two prominent examples of first-line treatment are the glucose transporter 1 (GLUT-1) deficiency and pyruvate dehydrogenase complex deficiency (PDCD) syndromes. GLUT-1 deficiency syndrome is a rare disorder in which the brain cannot get its necessary energy through glucose metabolites because they cannot cross the "blood-brain barrier." By maximizing the body's level of ketones in a controlled and healthy way through the use of the ketogenic diet, there is a new energy source made available to the brain so that it can function properly. Recent studies would suggest that the diet may not be a lifelong treatment for GLUT-1, and it could possibly be stopped in adolescence.

PDCD syndrome is a rare neurodegenerative disorder, usually starting in infancy, that is associated with abnormalities of the body's citric acid cycle. Proper production of carbohydrates is interfered with, and there is a resultant deficit in energy throughout the body, accompanied by a dangerous buildup of lactic acid. The result is damage to the brainstem.

In these two illnesses, the ketogenic diet acts as both an anticonvulsant treatment, as well as possibly treating other, nonepileptic, manifestations of the underlying metabolic derangement. Early consideration and confirmation of these two diagnoses offers the possibility of avoiding all or at least some of the devastating lifetime developmental condition resulting from a disease, injury, or other trauma.

The evidence is certainly less clear when consideration of the ketogenic diet as primary therapy is expanded to other epilepsy types and syndromes known as age-dependent/age-specific epileptic brain disorders. Examples are Ohtahara syndrome (early infantile epileptic encephalopathy with burst suppression), which is frequently associated with central nervous system malformation; West syndrome with infantile spasms, hypsarrhythmia EEG pattern, developmental arrest and/or regression; Lennox-Gastaut syndrome with slow spike-wave on EEG and multiple seizure types; early-onset myoclonic epilepsy frequently associated with metabolic abnormalities; migrating partial epilepsy of infancy; and Dravet syndrome (severe myoclonic epilepsy in infancy) with atypical early onset febrile seizures that become intractable mixed seizures and are associated with the SCNA-1 gene mutation in 40% of cases.

West syndrome is the most studied and there is lots of information that in about half of children who are started on the diet, about 90% of the spasms may go away. What is most interesting is that the sooner the diet is started the better the outcome. Knowing this, why not use it first? We have done that—data from our center show that there is no difference in the time it takes to seizure freedom comparing treatment with the "gold standard" adrenocorticotrophic hormone (ACTH) versus the ketogenic diet. While the EEG improved and normalized faster with ACTH at 1 month in spasm-free babies, there was no difference at 2–5 months. Most significantly, the incidence of side effects was lower in the babies treated with the ketogenic diet, as well as the risk of the spasms coming back. We now use the ketogenic diet routinely here at Johns Hopkins as a first-line therapy.

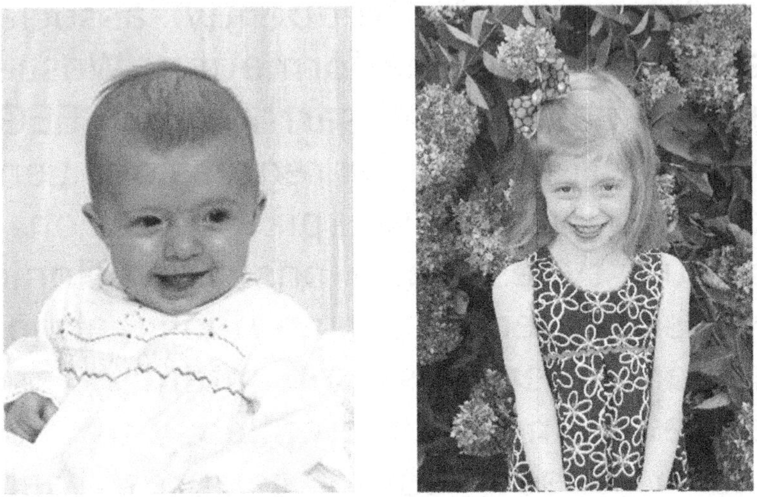

FIGURE 24.1 and 24.2 Carson Harris, one of our babies with new-onset infantile spasms treated with the diet alone, at 6 months when she developed spasms and today, now normal (see Chapter 13 for more information about The Carson Harris Foundation). Courtesy of The Carson Harris Foundation.

These are severe, early-onset epilepsies that have gotten the attention of ketogenic diet centers, but early therapeutic intervention has been restricted by the belief that the ketogenic diet is unsafe for use in newborns and infants. Data published 15 years ago reported that the infant brain was four times more efficient than the adult brain in extracting and utilizing ketone bodies. In 2001, in a retrospective study summarizing the experience treating 32 infants under age 24 months, it was concluded that "the ketogenic diet should be considered safe and effective treatment for infants with intractable seizures." Additional publications show that the side-effect profiles of ketogenic diet use in very young children do not differ significantly from older children, which should lead doctors to increased consideration of the diet in this population. All these "catastrophic" epilepsy syndromes of infancy merit controlled studies to determine which are most likely to respond to initial or early ketogenic diet treatment as opposed to anticonvulsant medications.

There is also recently published research that reviews the usefulness of the ketogenic diet in status epilepticus, an acute life-threatening state where the brain is in a persistent state of continuous seizures. Early use of the ketogenic diet administered via gastric-tube (g-tube) feeding may be a rational therapy in certain specific febrile-seizure status states in school-aged children (the FIRES syndrome). Seizures from tuberous sclerosis complex and Rett disorder are very difficult to manage with medication, and there appears to be a role for very early use of ketogenic diet therapy once those diagnoses are confirmed and seizures begin.

Doose syndrome is an epilepsy syndrome of early childhood that is often resistant to medication and where the ketogenic diet offers a combination of virtually immediate seizure relief and long-term control. The Doose syndrome clinical and EEG pattern is clearly recognizable, and although up to this point in time medications are being used initially, the ketogenic diet allows the rapid discontinuation of medications, with seizure freedom even when the diet is stopped after 2 years. Multiple studies have shown that the diet is the *best* treatment for this condition, and nearly all these articles comment at the end that it should be considered "sooner" than as a last resort. At our center, we will mention the diet as soon as the first visit and at times offer it before medications. However, if one drug fails, especially Depakote®, we will strongly push the diet as the next choice.

There are some barriers in the medical system to using the ketogenic diet first. First, dietitians and neurologists have to change their mindset about the diet and consider it an appropriate "emergency" treatment option. That means dropping everything to start the diet and not putting these children on a waiting list that might take months. Insurance companies may not agree as well, and families might have to accept a financial burden if that happens. Second, parents would have to give the diet a chance to work. Although data would suggest that for infantile spasms the diet works within a week or two, in our experience the family is often very impatient if there is no benefit within days. The family would also have to understand that if the diet did *not* work, then they'd have to stop and move on to medications (especially for West syndrome where time is of the essence). Lastly, the education process for starting the diet would have to be shortened and streamlined. If not, a 4-day admission for education would certainly seem much more difficult than a 1-minute signing of a prescription. This book may help, along with the Internet and other resources, but the diet will need to be made easier and quicker for sure.

What is clear is that in 2011, the ketogenic diet is not an appropriate "last resort." Even if it is not being used first, it should be mentioned earlier in the treatment of epilepsy, certainly after two drugs have failed. By the time the 6th edition of this book is published eventually, we suspect the diet will be widely used as a first-line therapy for many of the epilepsy conditions mentioned in this chapter.

CHAPTER TWENTY FIVE

Adults and Diets

Things are changing quickly in the ketogenic diet world, and the use of dietary therapy in adults is a primary example of that. When we published our 4th edition of this book, we devoted only two paragraphs to discussing this topic. Now there is a good bit more to say. This chapter was written primarily by James Rubenstein with the added advice of Dr. Mackenzie Cervenka, who heads our epilepsy diet center for adults.

In the 69 years that passed between the report of what happened to 100 adults treated at Mayo Clinic in 1930 and a paper from Jefferson University in Philadelphia reviewing results from treating 11 adults (later expanded to 26), there were no other studies published in English-language medical journals. This was probably due to an incorrect perception that the diet was ineffective for adults. The truth is, the results were similar—that is, in the earlier study, 56% of patients had greater than 50% decrease in seizures, and 12% became seizure free. In the later study from 1999, the numbers were 54% and 27%. Of more interest, those results match up closely with the results most ketogenic diet centers report in longer term studies in children, where we expect 10% of patients to be seizure free, 25% to have 90% decrease in seizures, and 50% to have greater than 50% decrease.

Which, of course, leads to the question, "Why aren't adults using the ketogenic diet more?" The current thought we hear most often is that doing the diet in adults (starting with teenagers over 17 years old) is just "too hard." Even in the rare instances where their physicians are aware of the potential benefits that the ketogenic diet offered, adults often are simply unwilling to try it because of "the severe lifestyle change" required—no fast food, limited alcohol, no high carb snacks, and so forth.

However, the introduction of the modified Atkins diet (MAD) by our group and of the Low Glycemic Index Treatment (LGIT) at Massachusetts General in Boston may have changed all that. We elaborate on how those diets are initiated and managed in Section IV, but suffice to say, the relative ease with which these two newer alternatives to creating ketosis can be implemented has changed things pretty dramatically for older patients.

We have learned a lot about the use of MAD in adults:

- Initiation is rapid, and adults will begin to respond quickly if they are going to respond at all (mean 5 days).
- Although the amounts of fluids, protein, and calories are unrestricted, it is very important for extra amounts of fat to be eaten daily.

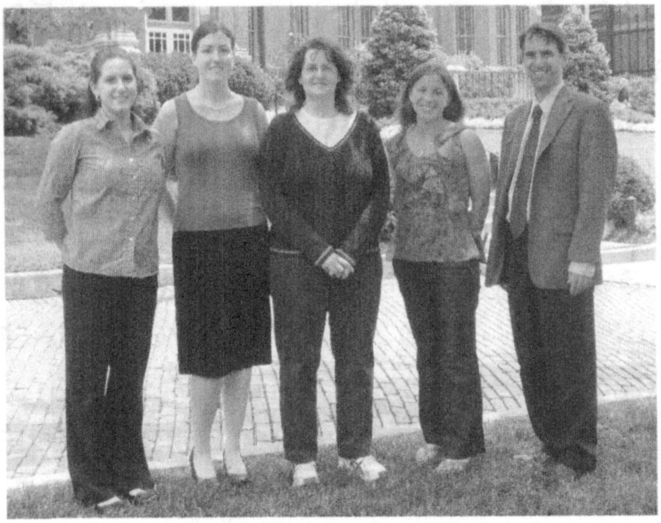

FIGURE 25.1 The Adult Epilepsy Diet Center team at Johns Hopkins Hospital.

- Adults can start at a slightly higher total carbohydrate allowance than children (20 grams versus 10 grams) and liberalize up to 25–30 grams after several months.
- Two months on MAD is likely a long enough trial on the diet to assess efficacy, as opposed to 3–6 months for children on the ketogenic diet.
- Lowering body mass index (BMI) and achieving weight loss both correlate with better response in adults, which is not true in children, when analyzed at 3 months. This may be due to compliance.
- Many adults who started the ketogenic diet as children can continue to do well when they are switched to the MAD.
- Cholesterol increases do occur; they need to be monitored and if changes in the types of fats don't

work, then a statin medication should be considered.

- Weight loss can occur—if it's planned, that's great.
- Kidney stones and constipation can occur, but risks can be lessened by staying hydrated.
- If adults are not seizure free, they often stop the diet (no matter how tough their seizures have been to control).

We are not the only center interested in the use of diets for adults. As of the writing of this chapter, 41 adults have tried the MAD (as documented in the literature). Forty-seven percent had a greater than 50% decrease in seizures by 3 months; many of whom felt better and had improved concentration. A very high proportion of adults who tried MAD these have complex partial seizure disorders, many of whom had prior placement of a vagus nerve stimulator (VNS) and previous intracranial epilepsy surgery before MAD was tried.

In August of 2010 we opened an Adult Epilepsy Diet Center here at Johns Hopkins. Dr. Mackenzie Cervenka is the medical director of the center (second from left in the photo above).

Another center opened in London in January of 2011 through Matthew's Friends. More and more epilepsy centers, neurologists, and dietitians are offering the diet to adults.

We anticipate treating increased numbers of patients as both they and their doctors learn about the potential benefits of a treatment previously thought to only be significantly beneficial to children. There are many unanswered questions about diets and adults, which may be solved by the next edition of this book:

- Do cholesterol increases lead to problems in adults who are on these diets for epilepsy?
- Is it safe during pregnancy? Is it perhaps even ideal for pregnancy (compared to anticonvulsants with known risks for birth defects)?
- Can it be done with limited dietitian support, knowing that many adult dietitians are not familiar or comfortable with treatment of epilepsy patients?
- Is the compliance issue really a problem, or can the diet be made easier?
- Should patients fast when starting the diet?
- How long should patients remain on the diet?
- Are there adults who are more likely than others to do better (e.g., certain kinds of seizures)?

CHAPTER TWENTY SIX

Diets and Other Neurologic Conditions

Although the ketogenic diet and perhaps even its alternative forms have now been accepted as treatments for epilepsy, new evidence suggests that ketogenic diets also may play a role in the treatment of some nonepileptic conditions, such as the following:

- Brain tumors and perhaps other cancers
- Severe head trauma and perhaps hypoxic/ischemic encephalopathy
- Stroke, heart disease
- Alzheimer's disease (AD)
- Parkinsonism
- Amyotrophic lateral sclerosis (ALS)
- Diabetes
- Autism
- Inflammatory disease
- Migraine
- Severe hyperactivity
- Other diseases

REMINDER: Use of the ketogenic diet in these conditions, as of this time, is anecdotal. This means that the diet has *NOT* as yet been established as a treatment for any of these conditions! However, there are promising leads or single case reports that suggest the ketogenic diets deserve further investigation for each of these conditions.

BRAIN TUMORS

Over many years, Dr. Thomas Seyfried and colleagues have studied the metabolism of tumors and of glial cells and neurons. They found that neurons and glial cells are able to metabolize ketone bodies as an alternative fuel to glucose, whereas tumor cells metabolize mainly glucose. Dietary restriction can lower glucose levels, and the ketogenic diet further lowers glucose levels—while also providing ketone bodies for neuronal metabolism. Caloric restriction and the ketogenic diet are also antiangiogenic (do not promote the growth of blood vessels need for tumor growth) as well as enhancing cell death. Because tumor cells require glucose and an increasing blood supply to provide glucose and oxygen and are unable to metabolize the ketone bodies produced on a hypoglycemic-ketotic diet, they die. These results were seen in mice with implanted tumors as well as in two children with inoperable brain tumors reported by Nebeling of tumor regression clearly deserve further study.

Seyfried and colleagues are proposing an approach to brain cancer management that exploits the ability of normal cells to utilize ketones at the expense of tumor cells which are glucose dependent. Such studies, while slow in coming, are in progress, and are promising. The report by Seyfried and by Zuccoli et al. are first steps.

Other studies have been ongoing, including one in Germany and another at Albert Einstein in New York City. As of yet, these results have not been released. We think this is one of the most promising "nonepilepsy" indications, but it does require oncologists to be interested and willing to try it.

SEVERE HEAD TRAUMA AND HYPOXIA

Traumatic brain injury (TBI) is common in both adults and children and often results in permanent neurologic conditions. The trauma causes multiple changes in the brain including swelling, bleeding, the release of neurotransmitters, and shifts in ions across cell membranes. An initial rapid increase in glucose metabolism is followed by a prolonged depression of glucose metabolism. This depression has led to the administration of glucose to TBI patients, but the resultant hyperglycemia only worsened the outcome. Dietary supplements have been largely ineffectual. Fasting or a ketogenic-like diet suppressed the hyperglycemia and in rodent experiments improves tissue preservation after trauma.

Mayumi L Prins, PhD, has questioned the current standards of glucose preservation after traumatic brain injury and has suggested using the ketogenic diet to lower glucose while providing alternative energy. Decreased cortical pathology and improved motor and cognitive performance has been seen in young rodents after TBI and starvation. Starvation and the administration of ketones—or the ketogenic diet—may be better than current treatments, at least in young children. Perhaps the same is true in the newborn after hypoxic-ischemic injury. Of course, it would certainly be best if the diet could be in place (and being eaten) before the trauma occurs, but that's another study.

ALZHEIMER'S DISEASE

This degenerative disease occurring in older individuals is characterized by progressive loss of memory. When Alzheimer's disease (AD) is suspected, the diagnosis is usually confirmed with behavioral assessments and cognitive tests. There is no curative treatment available at present.

There are suggestions that the ketogenic diet not only may provide symptomatic benefit but could have beneficial disease-modifying activity as well. This also may be true for a broad range of other brain disorders characterized by the death of neurons. In AD, it is said that high carbohydrate intake worsens the patient's cognitive performance and behavior. The ketogenic diet and caloric restriction affect beta-amyloid levels, the hallmark of AD in rodent models.

In 2009, a drug called Axona® was put on the market by a company called Accera, Inc. This is an

FDA-approved "medical food" that is caprylic triglyceride, a form of MCT oil. It is a once-daily powder that is designed to improve cognitive function in patients with Alzheimer's. The company Web site is www.about-axona.com. At this time it is too early to tell if this is really useful as studies are preliminary.

PARKINSON'S DISEASE AND ALS

Animal studies and anecdotal patient reports indicate that the ketogenic diet may modify and even reverse the manifestations of both Parkinson's disease and amyotrophic lateral sclerosis (ALS), but there are no published human studies to confirm these reports. An ongoing study of ALS is underway at Johns Hopkins and Cornell.

AUTISM AND AUTISTIC SPECTRUM DISORDERS

Autism is a disorder of neural development characterized by impaired social interaction and communication and by restricted and repetitive behaviors. The autistic spectrum disorders range in severity from pervasive developmental disorders to Asperger's syndrome. There is no specific treatment for these disorders to date. One pilot study of the ketogenic diet from Crete reported some improvements in some of the children.

Anecdotal reports of behavioral improvements in autistic children with seizures treated with the ketogenic diet also have appeared. Clearly, further study is indicated.

DIABETES

Diabetes is a condition in which a person has high blood sugar, either because the body does not produce enough insulin or because cells do not respond to the insulin that is produced. The elevated blood sugar (hyperglycemia) and the ketosis that may accompany it can cause shifts in metabolism resulting in diabetic ketoacidosis, which may result in coma and even death.

DIABETIC ketoacidosis is very different from the ketosis of the ketogenic diet. In the former, an individual has markedly elevated blood glucose in addition to the ketone bodies, the individual has acidosis as well as a depletion of potassium and fluids. Diabetic ketoacidosis is a medical emergency and can be fatal.

The ketosis associated with the ketogenic diet has elevated ketone bodies and a mild acidosis, but is *NOT* life threatening.

Before the discovery of insulin, diabetes was ultimately fatal, a result of ketoacidosis, and children with diabetes were expected to live less than 1 year. Starvation with a 450-calorie diet was one of the few forms of treatment. Another, devised by Frederick M. Allen, found that a diet with 70% fat and 8% carbohydrate could eliminate the sugar in the urine among hospitalized patients. Before the discovery of insulin this became one of the most common dietary treatments.

The discovery of insulin changed treatment. Unfortunately, warnings about the lethality of ketoacidosis have led to physicians' continuing disbelief that individuals can thrive while in ketosis. They do not understand the difference between diabetic ketoacidosis and ketosis.

SEVERE HYPERACTIVITY

It is believed that sugar makes children hyperactive and that it should be restricted in those with hyperactivity syndromes. There are reports of decreased activity in rodents on ketogenic diets, but only anecdotal reports of the beneficial effects of ketogenic and ketogenic-like diets in decreasing the hyperactivity and distractibility of children treated for seizures. There are no reports of controlled trials of ketogenic diets for hyperactivity, but such studies are needed.

PAIN AND MIGRAINE

Does the ketogenic diet have effects on pain and inflammation? One recent report states that this is the case in rats.

What about migraine headaches? Some older articles, and even one of the original textbooks on the ketogenic diet from Dr. Fritz Talbot in 1930, discuss the diet as possibly helpful for migraines. We studied eight teenagers with severe migraine at Johns Hopkins Hospital over several years in a prospective trial. Sadly, not only was the modified Atkins diet ineffective in helping their headaches, but most stopped it after a few months. It also was very difficult to get teens to agree to the trial.

OTHER DISEASES

Current rapid acceptance of the ketogenic diet and reports of its possible use in a multitude of diseases other than epilepsy are promising a far wider role for this diet and its modified partners. Clearly, as the uses of the ketogenic diet are discovered and its metabolic effects understood, perhaps we will even be able to replace the ketogenic diet with a pill. That will be a day of celebration!

SECTION VII

Appendices

APPENDIX A

Medications and Keto-Friendly Products

MEDICATIONS

- Nearly all anticonvulsants are now generic. As a result, some of the lists of "preferred" medications we used (including those given in the 4th edition of this book) are out-of-date and no longer valid. For example, zonisamide has about 20 different generic formulations, so it's impossible to know the carbohydrate contents of each! In general, IV is better than pills. Pills are better than liquid or chewable forms. However, ask your pharmacist.
- Carbohydrates are frequently used as fillers and flavor enhancers in medications.
- Even small amounts of carbohydrate found in medications can sometimes affect seizure control on the diet.
- Many over-the-counter and prescription medications are not available in sugar-free forms. (Some may be labeled "sugar-free" when they are very low in carbohydrate, but there still may be enough to affect ketosis in your child.)
- If you are unsure about the contents of a medication you should call your pharmacy and explain the situation, and they should be able to help.

- As a general rule, avoid any medications in syrup or elixir forms.
- Compounding pharmacies can make sugar-free forms of some medications.
- Talk to your doctor and pharmacist about giving IV forms of medications by mouth (may require dose adjustment, however).
- Antibiotics can be particularly difficult because almost all contain carbohydrate. Work with your pharmacy to find the form with the lowest carbohydrate content.
- Certain medications, such as antihistamines and antibiotics, can affect seizure control even if they do not contain carbohydrates.
- As a last resort, if a medication with carbohydrates must be given, you can add a small amount of butter or oil to make it ketogenic.

Commonly Used Medications

- Feverall® suppositories (0carb)—best option for fever, teething, headache, pain—you can buy them over the counter at a local drugstore.
- Diastat® suppositories (no carb)
- Tylenol Junior Strength Caplets®—traces of carbohydrate, but less than 1kcal per caplet, and young children may only need 1/2 of a tablet
- Diabetic Tussin DM®—no sorbitol, saccharin-based cough suppressant, expectorant—best option for

cough/cold liquid medication—the rest have tons of sorbitol!

- Miralax®—for constipation
- Benefiber®—for constipation
- Polycitra K® and Bicitra®—for kidney stones
- Augmentin®—adult capsules—0 carbohydrate antibiotic
- Saline nose spray
- Vicks® vapo rub
- Original Neosporin® first aid ointment
- Desitin® ointment (original—not creamy)
- Genasyme® infant drops—sacharrin-based simethecone drops for gas/bloating (like Mylicon® drops)—made by Goldline/Ivax (800-327-4114/305-575-6000)

KETO-FRIENDLY PRODUCTS

Sunscreens

Coppertone Sport®
Coppertone Oil Free®

Lotions

Johnson's Baby Oil®
Johnson's Soft Lotion®—24 hour moisture
Johnson's Creamy Baby Oil®

Curel® lotion—original
Lubriderm Seriously Sensitive Lotion®
Nivea Body Original Lotion®

Shampoos and Conditioners

Pantene Pro V Classic Clean Shampoo®
Pantene Pro V Classic Clean Conditioner®
Pantene Pro V 2 in 1—Shampoo plus Conditioner®
L'Oreal Kids Orange Mango Smoothie Shampoo®
L'Oreal Kids Grape Conditioner®
L'Oreal Kids Extra Gentle 2 in 1 Shampoo®—Burst of Watermelon (green bottle)
Johnson's No More Tangles Spray Detangler®
Baby Magic Gentle Hair and Body Wash®
Baby Magic Gentle Baby Shampoo®

Body Wash/Soaps

Dove Sensitive Skin Soap®
Dove Moisturizing Body Bar®
Dove Moisturizing Body Wash®—Sensitive Skin
Baby Magic Gentle Baby Bath®—Original Baby Scent

Lip Care

Vaseline®
Chapstick® Cherry Lip Balm

Toothpaste

Arm and Hammer Original Paste®—best choice
Arm and Hammer Advance White®—best choice
Tom's of Maine®—peppermint or spearmint paste (trace sorbitol)

Baby Supplies

Baby Orajel Teething Swabs® (no sorbitol)
Desitin Ointment®—(original—not the creamy version)
Johnson's No More Tangles Spray Detangler®
Johnson's Baby Oil®
Johnson's Soft Lotion®—24-Hour Moisture
Johnson's Creamy Baby Oil®
Baby Magic Gentle Hair and Body Wash®
Baby Magic Gentle Baby Shampoo®
Baby Magic Moisturizing Baby Lotion®—powder scent
Baby Magic Gentle Baby Bath®—original baby scent

Extracts

McCormick®—Pure Almond, Pure Lemon, Pure Orange, Pure Pepper mint, Pure Anise

Bickford®—This company makes many keto-friendly extracts, including vanilla. Their number is included on your phone number list. When you call them to order, tell them that you are looking for pure extracts with no carbohydrate added.

Sweeteners

Liquid Sweet & Low®

Liquid Sweet 10®

Saccharin grains—but you must dissolve them in hot water prior to adding to foods/drinks!

Stevia® Pure Extract (liquid)—can be ordered via the Internet

Don't use large quantities of powder forms of sweeteners, because they contain carbohydrates!

Deodorant

Secret Solid®—Powder Fresh Scent

Foods and Products Used Often

Bickford Laboratories, Inc. (flavorings)
Toll free 1-800-283-8322
www.bickfordflavors.com

Canfield Diet Soda® (Diet Chocolate Fudge, Diet Cherry Chocolate, and Diet Swiss Crème)
847-604-8745 X4

Dukes Mayonnaise®
www.dukesmayo.com
1-888-339-2477

George's Aloe Vera® (for constipation)
281-240-2563

GLACEAU® (Fruit Water and Smart Water beverages without artificial sweeteners)
Toll free 1-800-746-0087 for distributors in your area

Hawaiian Ice Sno Maker® (sold at Target)
801-572-1982

Just the Cheese™ (baked cheese snacks)
Toll free 1-800-367-1711
www.specialcheese.com

Davinci Gourmet: Sugar Free Syrups
www.davincigourmet.com

Miracle Noodles®:
www.miraclenoodle.com

Konjac Shiratake®
www.konjacfoods.com

FORMULAS AND COMPONENTS

Ketocal®3:1 and 4:1
Nutritica North America
800-365-7354
www.shsna.com/pages/ketocal.htm
A consent form is needed from the dietitian prior to ordering.

RCF: Ross Carbohydrate Free®
Abbott Nutrition
http://abbottnutrition.com/products/products.aspx?pid=77

Microlipid®
Nestle Nutrition

www.nestle-nutrition.com/products

Polycose®
Abbott Nutrition
http://abbottnutrition.com/products/products.asp x?pid=276

MCT Oil

1. Nestle Nutrition: www.nestle-nutrition.com
2. Sci Fit MCT Oil® (multiple Web sites)
3. Smart Basics MCT Oil®: http://www.vitacost.com /Smart-Basics-MCT-Oil

VITAMINS AND MINERALS

Nano VM® 1–3 and 4–8
www.solacenutrition.com

Sugar-Free Bugs Bunny® or Scooby Doo®
http://oneaday.com/products/OAD_kids/bugs_co mplete/index.html

Calcium and Vitamin D
www.naturemade.com

Centrum New Formula®
www.centrum.com/product_detail_home.aspx?pr oductid=CENTRUM

SCALES

Ohaus Corporation
1-800-526-0659
www.ohaus.com

Pelouze Scale Company
1-800-638-3722
www.healthometer.com

COMPOUNDING PHARMACIES

Professional Compounding Centers of America, Inc.
To find a compounding pharmacy near you call:
1-800-331-2498
www.pccarx.com

The following are compounding pharmacies that we have used:

H&B Drugs
N. Arlington, NJ
Toll free 1-888-383-2010
Fax 201-997-8488
http://www.hbpharmacy.com/

Professional Arts Pharmacy
Baltimore, MD
1-800-832-9285

Fax 410-788-5686

APPENDIX B

Sample Letter of Medical Necessity for Ketogenic Diet Formulas

TO:
Case Review Services
Re: Ketogenic Diet Therapy
For: _____
DOB: _____

Attention Case Manager:

_____ is a _____-month-old boy/girl with a diagnosis of _____ and an intractable seizure disorder. (His/Her) seizures were occuring _____ times each day despite attempts at seizure control with _____ (name anticonvulsants here).

The ketogenic diet is a high fat, adequate protein, low carbohydrate formula that is individually calculated and prescribed to produce adequate ketosis to suppress the child's seizures. The formula, which is fed by (bottle/gastrostomy tube), comprises _____. The formula must be supplemented with multivitamins and minerals in order to be nutritionally complete.

We are requesting that, because these components constitute an antiepileptic therapy rather than just a nutritional formula, they be covered under your policies.

Thank you for helping______to develop as free of seizures and medications as possible.

Sincerely,
XXX

APPENDIX C

Atkins Carbohydrate Gram Counter

The Atkins Carbohydrate Gram Counter is from *Dr. Atkins' New Diet Revolution 2002,* reproduced with permission of Atkins Nutritionals, Inc.

CARBOHYDRATE GRAM COUNTER

FOOD	CARBOHYDRATE GRAMS
MILK PRODUCTS	
Cream (light, 1 tbsp)	0.6
(sour, 2 tbsp)	1.0
(heavy, 1 tbsp)	0.5
Half and Half (1 tbsp)	0.7
Milk (whole, 1 cup)	11.0
(soy, unsweetened, 1 cup)	13.0
Plain Yogurt (skim, 1 cup)	13.0
(whole, 1 cup)	12.0
CHEESE	
American (1 oz)	0.5
Camembert (1 oz)	0.5
Cheddar (1 oz)	0.6
Cottage (fat-free, 1 cup)	10.0
(whole, 1 cup)	8.0
Cream Cheese (2 tbsp)	1.0
Feta (1 oz)	1.0
Muenster (1 oz)	1.0
Provolone (1 oz)	1.0
Swiss (1 oz)	0.5
NUTS	
Almond Paste (1 oz)	14.5
Almonds (1 oz)	5.5
Brazil (1 oz)	3.1
Cashews (1 oz)	8.3
Coconut (1 oz)	4.3
Hazelnuts (filberts) (1 oz)	4.7
Macadamia (1 oz)	4.5
Peanut Butter (1 tbsp)	3.0
Peanuts (1 oz)	5.4
Pecans (1 oz)	4.1
Pignolia (1 oz)	3.3
Pistachio (1 oz)	5.4
Pumpkin Seeds (1 oz)	4.2
Sesame Seeds (1 tbsp)	1.4
Soybeans (½ cup)	6.0
Sunflower Seeds (1 oz)	5.6
Walnuts (1 oz)	4.2
GRAINS	
Bagel (1)	30.0
Bread (pumpernickel, 1 slice)	17.0
(whole wheat, 1 slice)	11.0
Corn Muffin	20.0
Farina (1 cup)	22.0
Frozen Waffle	29.0
Noodles (1 cup cooked)	37.3
Oatmeal (1 cup cooked)	27.0

FOOD	CARBOHYDRATE GRAMS
Pancake (using dry mix)	17.4
Popcorn (popped 1 cup)	5.0
Rice (cooked 1 cup)	49.6
(puffed 1 cup)	11.5
SOUPS	
Chicken Consommé (1 cup)	1.9
Chicken Gumbo (1 cup)	7.4
Cream of Chicken (1 cup)	14.5
Cream of Mushroom (1 cup)	16.2
Turkey Rice (1 cup)	10.0
HERBS	
Allspice (1 tsp)	1.4
Basil (1 tsp)	0.9
Caraway (1 tsp)	1.1
Celery (1 tsp)	0.6
Cinnamon (1 tsp)	1.8
Coriander Leaf (1 tsp)	0.3
Dill Seed (1 tsp)	1.2
Garlic Clove (1)	0.9
Ginger Root (fresh, 1 oz)	3.6
(ground, 1 tsp)	1.3
Saffron (1 tsp)	0.5
Tarragon (1 tsp)	0.8
Thyme (1 tsp)	0.9
Vanilla (double strength, 1 tsp)	3.0
VEGETABLES	
Asparagus (4 spears)	2.2
Beans, green (boiled, 1 cup)	6.8
Beans, yellow or wax (boiled, 1 cup)	5.8
Broccoli (1 cup)	8.5
Brussels Sprouts (1 cup)	9.9
Cabbage (1 cup)	6.2
Carrot (7 in.)	7.0
Cauliflower (1cup)	5.1
Celery (1 stalk)	1.6
Coleslaw (1 cup)	8.5
Collards (1 cup)	9.8
Corn (1 ear, 5 in.)	16.2
Cucumber (sliced, 1 cup)	3.6
Dandelion (1 cup)	6.7
Endive (1 cup)	2.1
Kale (1 cup)	6.7
Kohlrabi (1 cup)	8.7
Lettuce (Romaine, 1 cup)	1.9
(Boston, 1 cup)	1.4
(Iceberg, 1 cup)	1.6

FOOD	CARBOHYDRATE GRAMS
Mushrooms (1 cup)	3.1
Mustard Greens (1 cup)	5.6
Okra (1 cup)	9.6
Onion (1 cup)	14.8
Parsley (1 tbsp)	0.3
Parsnips (1 cup)	23.1
Peas (1 cup cooked)	19.4
Peppers (green, 1 cup)	7.2
(red, dried, 1 tsp)	1.4
Potato (baked, 1)	32.8
Potato Salad (1 cup)	33.5
Pumpkin (3½ oz)	7.0
Radish (large, 10)	2.9
Spinach (1 cup)	6.5
Squash (summer, 1 cup)	6.5
(winter, 1 cup)	25.5
Sweet Potato (baked, 1)	37.0
Tomato (raw 2½ in.)	5.8
(cooked, 1 cup)	13.3
(juice, 1 cup)	10.4
Turnips (cooked, 1 cup)	11.3
(greens, 1 cup)	5.2
PROTEIN (FAT OR LEAN, WITHOUT BREADING)	
Fish, Poultry, Meat or Eggs	0-trace
FATS/OILS	
Olive, Canola, Safflower, etc.	0-trace
BEANS	
Black-eyed (1 cup)	38.0
Lima (1 cup)	33.7
Navy (1 cup)	40.3
Red Kidney (1 cup)	39.6
Soybeans (1 cup cooked)	19.4
Split Peas (1 cup)	41.6
Tofu/Bean Curd (2-in. cube)	2.9
FRUIT	
Apple (1 medium, 2¾ in.)	20.0
Applesauce (unsweetened, 1 cup)	26.4
Apricots (fresh, 3)	13.7
Avocado (California)	13.0
(Florida)	27.0
Banana (1)	26.4
Blackberries (1 cup)	18.6
Blueberries (1 cup)	22.2
Cantaloupe (½ melon, 5 in.)	20.4
Cherries (1 cup)	20.4
Grapefruit (pink, ½)	10.3
Grapes (10)	9.0

FOOD	CARBOHYDRATE GRAMS
Honeydew (1 cup)	13.1
Kiwi (1 medium)	9.0
Lemon	6.0
Lemon Juice (1 cup)	19.5
Mango (1 cup)	27.7
Olive (green, pitted)	2.5
Orange (1 medium)	16.0
Papaya (1 medium)	30.4
Peach (2½ in.)	9.7
Pear (3½ in.)	31.0
Pineapple (1 cup)	21.2
Plum (1 medium)	17.8
Prunes (1)	5.6
Raspberries (1 cup)	21.0
Rhubarb (cooked w/sugar, 1 cup)	97.2
Strawberries (1 cup)	12.5
SAMPLES OF CARBOHYDRATE "FATTENING" ITEMS	
Apple Pie (homemade, 1 slice)	61
Apple Turnover	30
Banana Split	91
Bean Burrito	48
Cheeseburger (¼ pounder)	33
Chicken Salad Sandwich	27
Cornbread Stuffing (½ cup)	69
Devil Dog	30
Egg Roll (1)	30
French Toast (2 slices)	34
Graham Crackers (1)	5
(chocolate covered, 1)	8
Hard Candy, Gumdrops, Jelly Beans (1 oz)	25
Honey (1 oz)	34
Hot Dog with Bun (1)	24
Ice Cream Soda (1 cup)	49
Macaroni with Cheese (1 cup)	40
Onion Rings (fast food order)	33
Peanut Brittle (1 oz)	23
Pecan Pie (homemade, 1 slice)	41
Pizza (1 slice)	24
Popsicle	17
Rolled Oats (1 cup cooked)	23
Saltines (1)	2
Shake (medium)	90
Sherbet (lemon, ½ cup)	45
Soda Crackers (1)	4
Tapioca Cream (½ cup)	22
Toaster Pastry (frosted, blueberry)	34
Waffles (plain, homemade, 1)	28
Whaler	64
White Sugar (1 oz)	28

Courtesy of Atkins Nutritionals, Inc.

APPENDIX D

Physicians Providing the Ketogenic Diet Worldwide as of November 2010

Of note, this list was provided to me by child neurologists, parents, and dietitians and does not necessarily constitute endorsement of the particular ketogenic diet center. This list is continuously updated at www.epilepsy.com/epilepsy/keto_physicians Please ask your neurologist for more information!

Countries in grey shading offer the ketogenic diet.

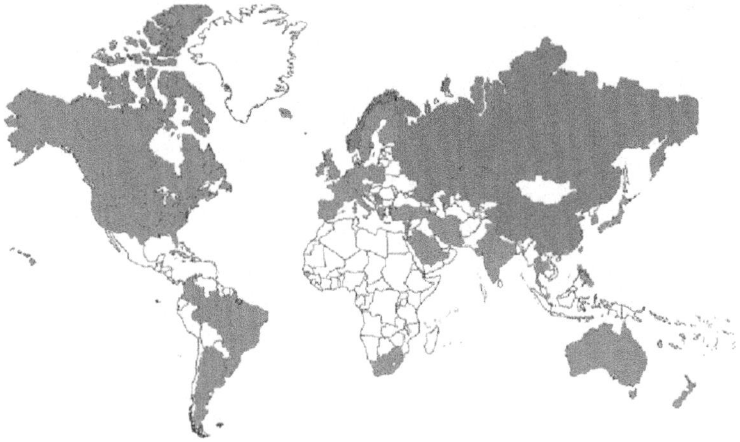

NORTH AMERICA*

[* *For centers in the United States (too many to count!), please go to* www.myketocal.com/findcenter .aspx]

Drs. Peter and Carol Camfield
Dalhousie University and the IWK Health Centre
PO Box 9700
Halifax, Nova Scotia
Canada, B3K 6R8
Phone: 902-470-8479
Fax: 902-470-8486

Dr. Elizabeth J. Donner
Division of Neurology
The Hospital for Sick Children
Dept of Neurology
555 University Ave
Toronto, ON M5G 1X8
Canada
Phone: 416-813-7037
Fax: 416-813-6334
Email: elizabeth.donner@sickkids.ca

Dr. Kevin Farrell
British Columbia Children's Hospital
4480 Oak Street
Room A303, Neurology
Vancouver, BC V6H 3V4
Canada
Phone: 604-875-2121
Fax: 604-875-2285
Email: kevin_farrell@telus.net

Drs. Daniel Keene and Sharon Whiting

Children's Hospital of Eastern Ontario
401 Smyth Rd
Ottawa, ON K1H 5L7
Canada
Phone: 613-523-5140
Fax: 613-523-2256
Email: dkeene@exchange.cheo.on.ca

Dr. Jeff Kobayashi
The Bloorview Macillan Children's Centre
25 Buchan Court
Toronto ON M2J 4S9
Canada
Phone: 416-425-6220 ext 6276
Fax: 416-753-6046
Email: jkobayashi@bloorviewmacmillan.on.ca

Dr. Anne Lortie
Hospital St. Justine
3175 Cote-Ste-Catherine
Montreal, PQ H3T 1C5
Canada
Phone: 514-345-4931
Fax: 514-345-4787
Email: lortie.a@sympatico.ca

Dr. Richard Tang-Wai
Stollery Children's Hospital
8440-112 Street
Edmonton, Alberta

Canada T6G 2B7
Phone: 780-407-1083
Email: Richard.Tang-Wai@capitalhealth.ca

Dr. Chais Calaña Gonzalez
Espec. Nutrition
Pediatric Hospital
Havana City
Cuba
Email: chaiscala@infomed.sld.cu

Dr. Pedro Marrero Martinez
University Hospital Juan Manuel Marquez
Calle E Nº517,
Esquina a 23
Apartamento 11-D
Vedado-Plaza
Havana City
Cuba
Phone: 05-2435205
Email: dpduran@infomed.sld.cu

SOUTH AMERICA

Dr. Roberto Caraballo
Hospital de Pediatría "Prof Dr Juan P Garrahan,"
Combate de los Pozos 1881,
C.P.1245
Buenos Aires
Argentina

Phone: 5411-4943-6116
Email: rhcaraballo@arnet.com.ar

Dr. Maria del Rosario
Hospital de Ninos
VJ Vilela
Rosario
Argentina
Phone: 54-341-480-8134
Email: mraldao@arnet.com.ar

Dr. Luis R. Panico
Hospital Vera Candiotti
Mendoza 3373
(3000) Santa Fe
Argentina
Phone/fax:+54-342-4558768
Email: dietasur@hotmail.com
http://usuarios.arnet.com.ar/mdemartini/index.htm

Dr. Beatriz Gamboni
Hospital de Ninos
Humberto Notti
Mendoza
Argentina
Phone: 54-261-496-1365
Email: bgamboni@nysnet.com.ar

Dr. Semprino Marcos
Clinica San Lucas

Neuquen
Argentina
Phone: 54-299-443-4730
Email: marcossemprino@yahoo.com

Dr. Sarisjulis Nicolas
Hospital de Ninos
Sor Maria Ludovica
La Plata
Argentina
Phone: 54-221-427-5115
Email: saris@lpsat.com

Dr. Maria Joaquina Marques-Dias
Professor of Neurology
University of São Paulo
Av Dr Eneas C Aguiar 647
05403-900 São Paulo, SP
Brazil
Phone: (11)3069-8673
Fax:(11)3069-8503
Email: majomadi@usp.br

Dr. Marcio M Vasconcelos
Av. das Americas, 700 sl 229 bl 6
Universidad Federal Fluminese
22640-100 Rio de Janeiro—RJ
Brazil
Phone: (55-21)2132-8080
Email: mmvascon@centroin.com.br

Dr. Ximena Raimann Tampier and Dr. Francesca Solari
Clinicas Las Condes
Lo Fontecilla 441
Santiago
Chile
Phone: 56-2-6108000
Email: xraimann@mi.cl

Dr. Andrea Avellanal
Hospital Británico
Benito Nardone 2217
11.300 Montevideo
Uruguay
Phone: 5982-711-91-86
Email: cinacina@adinet.com.uy

Dr. Luis Carlos Núñez López
Pediatric Neurologist
Carrera 29 # 47-108
Edificio Somes. Consultorio 20.
Bucaramanga
Colombia
Phone: 577-6475723
Fax: 577-6436124 extension 136
Email: lcnl007@intercable.net.co

Dr. Eugenia Espinosa
Hospital Militar Central
Bogota
Colombia

Phone: 0057-348-6868
Email: eugeniae@hotmail.com

Dr. Isaac Yepez
Hospital Pediatrico "Dr. Roberto Gilbert E."
Guayaquil
Ecuador
Phone: 005934-2287572
Email: iyepez@intramed.net

EUROPE

Dr. Martha Feucht
Universitatsklinik fur Neuropsychiatrie des Kindesund Jugendalters
Wahringer Gurtel 18-20
1090 Wien
Vienna
Austria
Phone:+43-40400-3012
Fax:+43-40400-2793
Email: martha.feucht@univie.ac.at

Dr. Barbara Plecko
University Klinik für Kinder-und Jugendheilkunde Graz
Auenbruggerplatz 30
A-8036 Graz
Austria
Phone:+43-316-385-82813
Fax:+43-316-385-2657

Email: barbara.plecko@meduni-graz.at

Prof. Wolfgang Sperl
Department of Pediatrics
Paracelsus Medical University
Salzburger Landeskliniken (SALK)
Müllner Hauptstraße 48
A-5020 Salzburg
Austria
Tel.: 0043-662-4482-2600
Fax: 0043-662-4482-2604
Email: w.sperl@salk.at

Dr. Lieven Lagae
Kinderneurologie—Epilepsie
Klinische Neurofysiologie
University Hospitals of Gasthuisberg
Herestraat 49
B-3000 Leuven
Belgium
Phone:+32-16-34-38-45
Fax:+32-16-34-38-42
Email: Lieven.Lagae@uz.kuleuven.ac.be

Nina Barisic, MD PhD
Professor of Pediatrics and Child Neurology
Department of Pediatrics
Division of Pediatric Neurology
Clinical Medical Center Zagreb
Zagreb medical school

Rebro, Kispaticeva 12
Zagreb, Croatia
Phone: 00-385-1-23-88-531
Fax: 00-385-1-24-21-894
Email: nina.barisic@zg.htnet.hr

Dr. Vladimir Komarek
Charles University Prague
2nd Medical School
Vuvalu 84, 150 06 Praha 5
Czech Republic
Phone:+420-2-2443-3302
Fax:+420-2-2443-3322
Email: Vladimir.komarek@lfmotol.cuni.cz

Dr. Maria Miranda
Danish Epilepsy Centre, Dianalund
Kolonivej 1
4293 Dianalund
Denmark
Phone: (+45)58271062
Email: MariMn@vestamt.dk

Dr. Peter Uldall
University Hospital of Copenhagen
Neuropaed clinic 5004
Rigshospitalet
Blegdamsvej
2100
Denmark

Phone:+4535455096
Fax:+4535456717
Email: peter.uldall@rh.hosp.dk

Dr. Elina Liukkonen
Helsinki and Vusimaa Hospital
Hospital for Children and Adolescents
PO Box 280
Finland
Phone: 011-358-9-4711-4711
Fax: 011-358-9-471-80-413
Email: elina.liukkone@hus.fi

Dr. Anne de Saint-Martin
Neuropédiatre
Service de Pédiatrie 1
CHU de Hautepierre
67098 Strasbourg Cedex
France
Phone: 33(0)388127734
Fax: 33(0)388128156
Email: anne.desaintmartin@chru-strasbourg.fr

Dr. Olivier Dulac
Hopital Saint Vincent de Paul
and Nadia Bahi-Buisson, MD, PhD
Service de Neuropédiatrie et Maladies Métaboliques
Hopital Necker Enfants Malades
149 Rue di Sevres
Paris 75743

France
Phone: 33-140-488111
Email: o.dulac@nck.ap-hop-paris.fr
and nadia.bahi-buisson@nck.ap-hop-paris.fr

Dr Stéphane Auvin
Service de Neurologie Pédiatrique et des Maladies Métaboliques
CHU Hôpital Robert Debré
48, boulevard Sérurier
75935 PARIS CEDEX 19
France
Phone:+33-1-40-03-57-07
Fax:+33-1-40-03-47-74
Email: auvin@invivo.edu

Dr. Laurence Lion Francois
Centre hospitalier Lyon Sud
Département de Neurologie pédiatrique
165 chemin du grand Revoyet
69 495 Pierre Bénite Cédex
France
Phone: 04-78-86-14-95
Fax: 04-78-86-57-16
Email: laurence.lion@chu-lyon.fr

Dr. Gia Melikishvili
Consultant Paediatric Neurologist
Children's Hospital
8 Lagidze Street

Tbilisi 0108
Georgia
Phone: 995-32-923429
Email: giam@caucasus.net

Dr. Birgit Walther
Teaching Hospital of the Charite
Humboldt University
Herzbergstrasse 79
D-10362 Berlin
Germany
Phone: 49-030-54723539
Fax: 49-0-30-54723502
Email: b.walther@keh-berlin.de

Dr. Adelheid Wiemer-Kruel
Ltd. Oberärztin Kinderklinik
Epilepsiezentrum Kork
Landstraße 1
77694 Kehl-Kork
Tel.: 07851/84-2230
Fax: 07851/84-2553
email: awiemer@epilepsiezentrum.de

Dr. R. Madeleyn
Filderklinik—Kinderabteilung
Im Haberschlai 7
D-70794 Filderstadt
Germany
Phone:+49-711-7703-0

Fax:+49-711-7703-1380
Email: t.reckert@filderklinik.de
www.filderklinik.de

Dr. Joerg Klepper
Aschaffenburg Children's Hospital
Am Hasenkopf
63739 Aschaffenburg
Germany
Phone:++49/6021/32-3601
Fax:++49/6021/32-3699
Email: joerg.klepper@klinikumaschaffenburg.de

Dr. Friedrich Ebinger
Dep. Pediatric Neurology
Children´s Hospital
University of Heidelberg
Im Neuenheimer Feld 430
69120 Heidelberg
Germany
Phone: 49.6221.56-8488
Fax: 49.6221.56-5744
Email: friedrich.ebinger@med.uni-heidelberg.de

Prof. Dr. F.A.M. Baumeister
Leiter Neuropädiatrie
Klinik für Kinder-und Jugendmedizin
Klinikum Rosenheim
Pettenkoferstr. 10
83022 Rosenheim

Germany
Tel.: 49-(0)8031-36-3457
Fax: 49-(0)8031-36-4927
Email: friedrich.baumeister@kliro.de

Dr. Athanasios Evangeliou
4th Pediatric Clinic of the
Aristotelian University of Thessaloniki
Papageorgiou Hospital
Ring Road
TK 56403
Thessaloniki
Greece
Phone:+30-2310-693920
Email: aeevange@auth.gr

Dr. Argirios Dinopoulos
University of Athens
Attico University Hospital
Athens
Greece
Phone:+30-2105831269
Fax:+30-2105832229
Email: argidino@yahoo.com

Dr. Thanos Covanis
Neurology Department
The Childrens Hospital "Agia Sophia"
Thivon and Levadis
11527, Athens

Greece
Phone:+302107751637
Email: graaepil@otenet.gr

Dr. Viktor Farkas
University Children's Hospital,
Semmelweis Medical School, Budapest
Bókay 53.
H-1083 Budapest
Hungary
Email: klissz@yahoo.de

Dr. Yr Sigurdardottir
Icelandic diagnostic center
Digranesvegi 5
200 Kopavogur
Iceland
Phone: (354)510-8400
Fax: (354)510-8401
Email: yr@greining.is

Drs. Bryan Lynch and Aisling Myers
The Childrens University Hospital
Temple Street
Dublin 1
Ireland
Phone: 00-353-86-8197831
Email: aislingmyers@hotmail.com

Dr. Giangennaro Coppola

Clinic of Child Neuropsychiatry
Second University of Naples Italy
Phone: 0039-81-5666695
Fax: 0039-81-5666694
Email: giangennaro.coppola@unina2.it

Dr. Federico Vigevano
Department of Neurology
Bambino Gesù Children's
Hospital 00165 Rome
Phone: 0039-06-68592262
Fax: 0039-06-68592463
Email: vigevano@opbg.net

Prof. Pierangelo Veggiotti
Dipartimento di Clinica
Neurologica e Psichiatrica
dell'Età Evolutiva
Laboratorio EEG dell'età
evolutiva
Fondazione "Istituto Neurologico
Casimiro Mondino"
Via Ferrata 6—27100—Pavia
Italy
Phone:+39-0382-380.344
Fax:+39-0382-380.286
Email: pveggiot@unipv.it

Dr. Volpi Lilia
Ausl Bo

Bellaria Hospital—Neurology
Bologna
Italy
Phone:+39-0516225111
Email: lilia.volpi@ausl.bo.it

Dr. Diana Fridrihsone and Dr. Jurgis Strautmanis
Children's University Hospital
Vienibas gatva 45
Riga LV 1004
Latvia
Phone:+371-29832436
Email: diana.fridrihsone@inbox.lv
Email: jurgis.strautmanis@eeg.lv

Dr. Jurgita Grikiniene
Vilnius University Children's Hospital
Santariskiu st.4
Vilnius, LT-08406
Lithuania
Phone:+370-68411405
Fax:+370-52720283
Email: jurgita.grikiniene@mf.vu.lt

Dr. Paul Augustijn
Observatie Kliniek voor Kinderen "Primula"
S.E.I.N.

Postbus 540
2130 AM Heemstede
The Netherlands
Phone: 31(0)23-558800
Fax: 31(0)23-558229
Email: paugustijn@sein.nl

Elles van der Louw (dietitian)
Erasmus MC-Sophia
UMC Utrecht Wilhelmina's
Childrens Hospital
PO Box 2060
Room sp2434
3000 CB Rotterdam
The Netherlands
Phone: 003110-4636290

Dr. Björn Bjurulf
Ullevål University hospital
0407 Oslo
Norway
Phone: 47-22118080
Fax: 47-22118663
Email: bjorn.bjurulf@ulleval.no

Dr. Anna Bremer
National Centre of Epilepsy
Pb.53, 1306 Basum post-terminal
Oslo
Norway

Phone: 47-67501000
Email: anna.bremer@epilepsy.no
Kathrine Haavardsholm RD
Email: Katherine.c.haavardsholm@epilepsy.no

Dr. Maria Zubiel
Dept. of Child Neurology
Institute of Polish Mother
Memory Hospital
93-338 Lodz, Rzgowska 281/289
Poland
Phone: 004842-2712080
Fax: 004842-2711412
Email: mzubiel@op.pl

Dr. Sergiusz Jozwiak
Professor and Head, Pediatric
Neurology
The Children's Memorial Health
Institute
Al. DZieci Polskich 20
04-736 Warszawa
Poland
Phone: 4822-8153417
Fax: 4822-8157402
Email: jozwiak@czd.waw.pl

Dr. Magdalena Dudzinska
Chorzowskie Centrum Pediatrii i Onkologii
Ul. Truchana 7

41-005 CHORZOW
Poland
Phone: 032-34-90-005
Email: duzinska@chcpio.pl or mdudzinskapl@yahoo.c
om

Ana Faria RD and Conceição
Robalo MD
Hospital Pediátrico de Coimbra
Avenida Bissaya Barreto
3000 Coimbra
Portugal
Phone: 351-239-480-606
Fax: 351-239-480-315
Email: anafaria@chc.min-saude.pt

Dr. Sergey Aivazyan
Head of Child Neurology
The Child Moscow Research
Hospital
Aviatorov Street, 38
SoIntsevo
Moscow
Russia
Phone: (095)4521022,
+79166204051
Email: abc1231961@mail.ru

Dr. Lesley Nairn
Consultant Paediatrician

Royal Alexandra Hospital
Paisley
Scotland
Phone: 0141-580-4460
Email: Lesley.Nairn@rah.scot.nhs.uk

Dr. Bosanka Jocic-Jakubi
Nis Medical University School
Bul. Zorana Dindica 48
18000 Nis
Serbia
Phone:+381-18-238-706
Email: bosajj@yahoo.com

Dr. Nebojsa J. Jovic
Clinic of Neurology and
Psychiatry for Children and
Youth
Dr Subotica 6a Street
11 000 Belgrade Serbia
Phone:+381-11-2658-355
Fax:+381-11-64-50-64
Email: njjovic@eunet.yu

Dr. David Neubauer
Department of Child, Adolescent & Developmental
Neurology
University Childrens' Hospital
Vrazov trg 1
1525 Ljubljana

Slovenia
Phone:+386.1.5229.273
Fax:+386.1.5229.357
Email: david.neubauer@mf.uni-lj.si

Dr. J. Campistol
Cap Servei de Neurologia
Hospital Sant Joan de Déu
Passeig Sant Joan de Déu, 2
08950-Esplugues (Barcelona).
Spain
Phone: 93-2532153
Fax: 93-2033959
Email: campistol@hsjdbcn.org

Dr. Antonio Gil-Nagel
Servicio de Neurología
Programa de Epilepsia
Hospital Ruber Internacional
La Masó 38, Mirasierra
28034 Madrid
Spain
Phone: 0034-913875250
Fax: 0034-913875333
Email: agnagel@ya.com

Dr. Per Amark and Dr. Maria
Dahlin
Astrid Lindgrens Childrens
Hospital

Karolinska Hospital
S-171 76 Stockholm
Sweden
Phone:+46-8-5177-7026
Fax:+46-8-5177-7608
Email: per.amark@ks.se

Dr. Tove Hallbook
University Hospital
Se-221 85 Lund
Sweden
Phone: 46-46-17-1000
Fax: 46-46-14-5459
Email: tove.hallbook@telia.com

Dr. Isa Lundstrom
Department of Pediatrics
Nordland University Hospital
SE-901 85 Umeå
Sweden
Email: isa.lundstrom@bredband.net

Dr. Oswald Hasselmann
Neuropediatrics
Ostschweizer Kinderspital
Claudiusstrasse 6
CH-9006 St. Gallen
Switzerland
Phone:+41(0)71-243-7-363 bzw.-111
Email: oswald.hasselmann@gdkispi.sg.ch

Dr. Gabriela Wohlrab
University Children's Hospital,
Neurophysiological Department,
Steinwiesstrasse 24,
CH-8032 Zürich
Switzerland
Phone: 0041-1-266-77-01
Email: Gabriele.Wohlrab@kispi.unizh.ch

Dr. Meral Topcu
Prof. of Pediatrics and Pediatric
Neurologist
Hacettepe Children's Hospital
Dept. of Child Neurology
06100 Ankara
Turkey
Phone: 90-312-3051165
Fax: 90-312-4266764
Email: mtopcu@hacettepe.edu.tr

Dr. Helen Cross
Reader and Honorary Consultant
in Paediatric Neurology
Institute of Child Health and
Great Ormond Street
Hospital for Children NHS Trust
The Wolfson Centre
Mecklenburgh Square
London WC1N 2AP
UK

Phone: 44-207-813-8488
Fax: 44-207-829-8627
Email: h.cross@ich.ucl.ac.uk

Dr. Colin Ferrie
Department of Paediatric
Neurology
Clarendon Wing
Leeds General Infirmary
Leeds LS2 9NS
UK
Phone: 0113-392-2188
Fax: 0113-392-5731
Email: Collin.Ferrie@leedsth.nhs.uk

Dr. Frances Gibbon
Department of Child Health
University Hospital of Wales
Cardiff
UK
Phone: 44-29-2074-3542
Email: Frances.Gibbon@cardiffandvale.wales.nhs.uk

Dr. Jayaprakash A Gosalakkal
Consultant Paediatric Neurologist
University Hospitals of Leicester
CDC/Windsor LRI
Leicester LE1 5WW
UK
Phone: 011441162585564

Fax: 011442587637
Email: Jay2world@aol.com

Dr. Sunny George Philip
Consultant Paediatric Neurologist
Birmingham Childrens Hospital
Birmingham
UK
B4 6NH
Phone: 011441213338149
Fax: 011441213338151
Email: SUNNY.PHILIP@bch.nhs.

Dr. Timothy Martland
Consultant Paediatric Neurologist
The David Lewis Centre
Mill House, Warford
Near Alderley Edge
Cheshire SK9 7UD
UK
Phone:+44-161-727-2346
Email: Timothy.Martland@CMMC.nhs.uk

Dr Ruth E Williams
Consultant Paediatric Neurologist
Evelina Childrens Hospital
Guy's and St Thomas' NHS Foundation Trust
Lambeth Palace Road
London SE1 7EH
UK

Phone:+44-207-188-3998
Fax:+44-207-188-0851
Email: Ruth.Williams@gstt.nhs.uk

Dr. Ruby Schwartz
Central Middlesex Hospital
Acton Lane
London NW10 7NS
UK
Phone: 020-8453-2121
Fax: 020-8453-2096
Email: Ruby.Schwartz@nwlh.nhs.uk

Dr. Neil H. Thomas
Consultant Paediatric Neurologist
Southampton University Hospitals NHS Trust
Southampton General Hospital
Mailpoint 021
Tremona Road
Southampton SO16 6YD
UK
Phone:+44-23-8079-4457
Fax:+44-23-8079-4962
Email: neil.thomas@suht.swest.nhs.uk

MIDDLE EAST

Hameeda Hamad Al-Shammari RD
Kuwait Hospital for Children
Kuwait

Email: h.dietitian98@hotmail.com

Dr. Mohammad Ghofrani
Professor of Paediatric Neurology
Shaheed Beheshti University of Medical Sciences and Health Services:
Mofid Hospital
Shariati St.
Tehran
Iran
Phone: 98-21-22200041

Dr. Bruria Ben'Zeev
Safra Children's Hospital
Sheba Medical Center
Ramat Gan
Israel 52621
Phone: 97235302577
Email: benzeev4@netvision.net.il

Dr. Eli Heyman
Asaf Harofe Medical Center,
Tel Aviv University
Zerifin 70300
Israel.
Phone:00972-8-9778466
Email: eheyman@post.tau.ac.il

Dr. Tally Lerman-Sagie
Director of Pediatric Neurology Unit

Wolfson Medical Center
Holon
Israel
Phone: 97235028458
Fax: 97235028141
Email: asagie@post.tau.ac.il

Dr. Generoso G. Gascon
Dept. of Neuroscience, MBC J-76
King Faisal Specialist Hospital & Research Center
P.O. Box 40047 Jeddah 21499
Saudi Arabia
Phone:+(966-2)667-7777, Ext.5813
Fax:+(966-2)667-7777, Ext.5819
Email: generoso_gascon@hotmail.com

Mouaz Al-Sbei, MD
Head of Neurology Section
International Medical Center
P.O. Box 2172 Jeddah 21451
Saudi Arabia
Phone:+966-2-650-9000 ext: 4712
Fax:+966-2-650-9001
Email: msbei@imc.med.sa

Dr. Adel A.H. Mahmoud
Consultant Pediatric Neurologist
Pediatric Neurology Department, Neuroscience Center
King Fahad Medical City
Riyadh

Saudi Arabia
POB 365814, Post Code 11393
Email: amahmoud@kfmc.med.sa

Dr. Mohammed Al-Malik and Ms. Unita Botes (dietitian)
Johns Hopkins—Tawam Hospital
PO Box 15258
Al Ain
United Arab Emirates
Phone: 971-3-767-7444
Email: mmalik@tawam-hosp.gov.ae

AFRICA

Dr. Tuschka du Toit
Registered Dietician
PO Box 4404
Rietvalleirand
South Africa 0174
Phone and Fax:+27-12-345-1392
Email: tuschka@absamail.co.za

Dr. Simon Strachan
Bedford gardens Hospital
Paediatric Centre
Bradford Road
Bedford gardens
Gauteng
South Africa
Phone: (011)493-2613/(011)622-2771

Email: sstracha@mweb.co.za
Email: megawlk@absamail.co.za

Dr. Jo M Wilmshurst
Head of Paed Neurology
5th Floor ICH
Department of Paediatrics
Red Cross Children's Hospital
Rondebosch
Cape Town 7700
South Africa
Fax: 027-21-689-2187
Email: wilmshur@ich.uct.ac.za

ASIA

Liao Jian Xiang, MD, PhD
Shenzhen Children's Hospital
China Medical University
7019 Yi Tian Road
Shenzhen, Guangdong Province
P R China 518026
Phone:+86-755-83936150
Fax:+86-755-83936148
Email: epilepsycenter@medmail.com.cn

Lai-Wah Eva Fung MRCP
Department of Pediatrics
30-32 Ngan Shing Street
Shatin, New Territories

Hong Kong Special Administrative Region
China
Phone: 852-2632-2981
Fax: 852-2636-0020
Email: eva_fung@cuhk.edu.hk

Winsy Leung RD
818 Health Professionals
Suite 818, Central Building
1 Pedder Street
Hong Kong
CHINA
Phone: 852-2526-6332
Email: winsyleung@children818.com

Dr. Chak Wai Kwong
Tuen Mun Hospital
Tsing Chung Koon Road
Tuen Mun, New Territories, Hong Kong
China
Phone: 852-2468-5111
Fax: 852-2456-9111
Email: chakwk@gmail.com

Dr. Ada Yung
Department of Paediatrics and Adolescence Medicine
University of Hong Kong
Queen Mary Hospital
Hong Kong SAR
Phone: (852)-2855-4485

Fax: (852)-2855-1523
Email: vcnwong@hkucc.hku.hk
Email: ayung@hkucc.hku.hk

Deng Yu Hong
Guangzhou Medical College
Chang-Gang-Dong Road 250
Guangzhou, Guangdong
PR China 510260
Phone:+86-20-34152244
Fax:+86-20-34153378
Email: Deng3251@yahoo.com.cn

Dr. Janak Nathan
Shushrusha Hospital
Ranade Road, Dadar W
Mumbai 400028
India
Phone: 091-22-24446615
Email: jsvpnat@hotmail.com
http://www.ketodietindia.org

Dr. Anaita Hegde
106 Doctor House
Opp. Jaslok Hospital
Peddar Road
Wadia Children's Hospital
Mumbai 400 026
India
Phone:+91-22-23517883

Fax:+91-22-23512922
Email: anaitahegde@hotmail.com

Ritu Sudhakar
Chief Dietitian
Dayanand Medical College & Hospital
Tagore Nagar, Ludhiana 141001
India
Email: sudhakar_ritu@rediffmail.com

Dr. Sheffali Gulati
Dr. Suvasini Sharma
Child Neurology Division
Department of Pediatrics
All India Institute of Medical
Sciences,
New Delhi 110029
India
Phone:+91-11-26593209
Fax:+91-11-26588641
Email: suvasinisharma@rediffmail.com
Email: sheffaligulati@gmail.com

Dr. Elisabeth Herini
Gadjah Mada University
Dr. Sardjito Hospital
J1. Kesehatan 1 Yogyakarta 55284
Indonesia
Phone: 62-274-561616
Fax: 62-274-583745

Email: herini_es@yahoo.com

Dr. Yukio Fukuyama
Child Neurology Institute
6-12-17-201 Minami-Shinagawa,
Shinagawa-ku
Tokyo 140-0004
Japan
Phone: 81-3-5781-7680
Fax: 81-3-3740-0874
Email: yfukuyam@sc4.so-net.ne.jp

Dr. Katsumi Imai
National Epilepsy Center, Japan
886 Urushiyama, Aoi Ward, Shizuoka City
Shizuoka, 420-8688
Japan
Phone:+81-54-245-5446
Fax+81-54-246-9781
Email: imaik@szec.hosp.go.jp

Dr. Tomohiro Kumada
Shiga Medical Center for Children
5-7-30 Moriyama
Moriyama City, Shiga, 524-0022
Japan
Phone:+81-77-582-6200
Email:tkumada@mccs.jp

Dr. Hirokazu Oguni

Dept of Pediatrics
Tokyo Women's Medical University
8-1 Kawada-cho, Shinjuku-ku
Tokyo 162-8666
Japan
Phone:+81-3-3353-8111
Fax:+81-3-5269-7338
Email: hoguni@ped.twmu.ac.jp

Dr. Benilda Sanchez
Head of the Epilepsy Monitoring Program of St. Luke's
Manila
Philippines
Phone: (632)723-0301 ext.5452
Fax: (632)727-5452
Email: beni779@hotmail.com

Dr. Derrick Chan Wei Shih
KK Women's and Children's Hospital
100 Bukit Timah Road
Singapore 229899
Phone: 065-6293-4044
Fax: 065-6394-1973
Email: Derrick.Chan.WS@kkh.com.sg

Dr. Hian-Tat Ong
Consultant, Paediatric Neurology and
Developmental Paediatrics
Children's Medical Institute
National University Hospital

Singapore
Phone: 065-67724391
Fax: 065-67797486
Email: OngHT@nuh.com.sg

Dr. Yong Seung Hwang
Professor, Pediatrics, Pediatric Neurology
Seoul National University Children's Hospital
28 Yon Gun Dong, Jong Ro Gu
Seoul, 110-744
South Korea
Phone: 82-2-760-3629
Fax: 82-2-743-3455
Email: childnr@plaza.snu.ac.kr

Dr. Heung Dong Kim
Associate Professor
Dept. of Pediatrics, Director in Child Neurology
Yonsei University College of Medicine, Severance Hospital
134, Shinchondong, Seodaemun-gu,
Seoul, 120-752
South Korea
Phone: 82-2-361-5511
Fax: 82-2-393-9118
Email: hdkimmd@yumc.yonsei.ac.kr

Dr. Huei-Shyong Wang
Division of Pediatric Neurology
Chang Gung Children's Hospital

Chang Gung University Taiwan
Phone: 886(0)968-110264
Fax: 886-3-3277295
Email: wanghs444@cgmh.org.tw

Dr. Pipop Jirapinyo
Professor of Pediatrics, Pediatric Nutritionist
Nutrition Unit
Department of Pediatrics
Faculty of Medicine Siriraj Hospital
Mahidol University
2 Prannok Road
Bangkoknoi, Bangkok 10700
Thailand
Phone: (662)411-2535
Email: sipjr@mahidol.ac.th

Dr. Pongkiat Kankirawatana
Director, Clinical Neurophysiology Lab
Pediatric Neurology, CHB-314
The Children's Hospital of Alabama
1600 7th Ave S.
Birmingham, AL 35233-1711
(information regarding Thailand experience)
Phone: 205-996-7850
Fax: 205-996-7867
Email: PKankirawatana@peds.uab.edu

AUSTRALIA/NEW ZEALAND

Dr. Deepak Gill
Paediatric Neurologist
Children's Hospital at Westmead
Cnr Hawkesbury Rd & Hainsworth St
Westmead
Sydney NSW 2145
Australia
Phone: 02-9845-2694
Fax: 02-9845-3905
Email: DeepakG@chw.edu.au

Dr. John Lawson
Child Neurologist
Sydney Children's Hospital
Sydney
Australia
Phone: 61-2-93821658
Fax: 61-2-93821580
Email: Lawson@sesahs.nsw.gov.au

Dr. Sophie Calvert
Staff Specialist in Paediatric Neurology
Neurosciences Department
Royal Children's Hospital
Herston
Australia
Phone: 07-3636-7487
Fax: 07-3636-5104

Email: Sophie_Calvert@health.qld.gov.au

Dr. Mark T. Mackay
Consultant Neurologist
Judy Nation (dietitian)
Department of Neurology
Royal Children's Hospital
Flemington Road, Parkville
Victoria 3052
Australia
Phone:+613-9345-5641
Fax:+613-9345-5977
Email: mark.mackay@rch.org.au
Email: judy.nation@rch.org.au

Dr. Lakshmi Nagarajan
Princess Margaret Hospital for Children
GPO Box D184
Perth WA 6840
Australia
Phone: (08)9340-8364
Fax: (08)9340-7063
Email: Lakshmi.Nagarajan@health.wa.gov.au

Dr. Thorsten Stanley
Senior Lecturer in Paediatrics
Wellington School of Medicine and Health Sciences
University of Otago
PO Box 7343 Wellington South
Wellington

New Zealand
Phone:+64-4-3855-999
Fax:+64-4-3855-898
Email: paedtvs@wnmeds.ac.nz

APPENDIX E

Modified Atkins Diet Sample Meals

Sunday Sample Meal

Breakfast

6oz decaffeinated coffee
1tbsp Half & Half cream
3 6-inch nitrate-free bacon slices
2 large scrambled eggs

Lunch

16 fluid oz water
7oz baked chicken breast
1/2 cup of romaine lettuce (loosely packed)
1/4 cup sliced cucumber (peeled)
2tbsp chopped raw mushrooms
1tbsp Italian dressing

Dinner

8 fluid oz diet soda
9oz salmon (grilled, broiled or baked)
3/4 cup steamed broccoli

1oz natural cheddar cheese (melt on broccoli)

Monday Sample Meal

Breakfast

6oz herbal tea
2 large fried eggs
2oz ham
2oz natural Swiss cheese

Lunch

12 fluid oz club soda
5 medium chicken wing pieces (not breaded)
2 medium celery stalks
1tbsp blue cheese dressing

Dinner

16 fluid oz water
7oz beef sirloin
1 cup romaine lettuce (loosely packed)
1/2 cup real bacon bits
1 large boiled egg
1tbsp Italian dressing

Remember to drink water throughout the entire day.

Sample Menu for Atkins Diet (15 Grams/Day)

	Sunday	Monday	Tuesday	Wednesday	Thursday	Friday	Saturday
Breakfast	Decaf coffee with Half & Half Bacon Scrambled Eggs	Herbal tea Ham and cheddar cheese omelet	Decaf coffee with Half & Half Sausage links Fried eggs	Decaf coffee with Half & Half Poached eggs Tomato with cheddar cheese	Water Vegetable and mozzarella cheese omelet with green peppers and mushrooms	Herbal tea Grilled ham steak Scrambled eggs with Cheddar cheese	Decaf coffee with Half & Half Steak and eggs
Lunch	Water Roast chicken breast Salad—Romaine lettuce, cucumber, mushrooms, and Italian dressing	Club soda Fried chicken wings Celery sticks Blue cheese dressing	Water Bunless double cheeseburger Lettuce Tomato Mayonnaise Dill pickle	Water Shrimp & scallops Steamed snow peas	Club soda Chicken Cobb salad—chicken breast, romaine lettuce, cucumber, boiled egg, and blue cheese dressing	Diet soda Sautéed beef and vegetables (green peppers and mushrooms)	Water Braised short ribs Salad—Romaine lettuce, tomato, alfalfa sprouts, and blue cheese dressing
Dinner	Diet soda Broiled salmon Steamed broccoli with cheddar cheese	Water Sirloin steak Salad—Romaine lettuce, bacon bits, 1 boiled egg, and Italian dressing	Diet Sprite Fried pork chops Buttered green beans	Diet soda Roasted turkey breast Spinach salad with mushrooms and Italian dressing	Water Seared tuna steak Steamed asparagus spears	Club soda Roast duck Steamed spinach	Water Grilled sea bass Steamed buttered cauliflower
Total Carbs	14.98 g	13.12 g	12.40 g	14.70g	13.95 g	14.78 g	14.84 g

APPENDIX F

Routine Ketogenic Diet Lab Studies for Children on the Diet

As part of our follow-up of the children on the ketogenic diet, you *must* obtain the following laboratory tests one (1) week prior to clinic visits. Please fill in your child's name and the date and have the neurologist fill in the rest.

KETOGENIC DIET LAB REQUEST (MUST FAST FOR MINIMUM OF 8 HOURS BEFOREHAND)

Patient Name: _____ Dx. Code: 345.01

Date: _____ Service or Clinic: Pediatric Epilepsy Center

Urinalysis

CBC with differential

Selenium level

Carnitine profile (total and free)

1,25-OH-Vitamin D level

(CMP-SMA20): to include chem panel-BUN, albumin

AST, creatinine, calcium, T. Bili, ALT, glucose, phosphorus, direct bilirubin, total protein, uric Acid, alkaline phosphatase

Complete Lipid Profile (fasting)

Anticonvulsant levels for these drugs:
[Space left intentionally blank in the original book]
Physician's Signature: _____ DEA # _____
Physician's Name (print): _____
PLEASE FAX RESULTS TO: _____

APPENDIX G

Selected References

GENERAL INFORMATION ON EPILEPSY

Freeman JM, Vining EPG, Pillas DJ. *Seizures and epilepsy in childhood.* 3rd edition. Johns Hopkins University Press, Baltimore, 2002.

REFERENCES ON THE EFFECTIVENESS AND ACCEPTABILITY OF THE KETOGENIC DIET

Farasat S, Kossoff EH, Pillas DJ, Rubenstein JE, Vining EP, Freeman JM. The importance of cognition in parental expectations prior to starting the ketogenic diet. *Epilepsy Behav* 2006;8:406–410.

Freeman JM, Kossoff EH. Ketosis and the ketogenic diet: 2010. *Adv Pediatrics* 2010;57:315–329.

Freeman JM, Vining EPG. Seizures rapidly decrease after fasting: preliminary studies of the ketogenic diet. *Arch Pediatr Adolesc* 1999;153:946–949.

Freeman JM, Vining EPG, Pillas DJ, Pyzik PL, Casey JC, Kelly MT. The efficacy of the ketogenic diet—1998: a prospective evaluation of intervention in 150 children. *Pediatrics*1998;102:1358–1363.

Gilbert DL, Pyzik PL, Vining EPG, Freeman JM. Medication cost reduction in children on the ketogenic diet: data from a prospective study of 150 children over one year. *J Child Neurol* 1999;14:469–471.

Hemingway C, Freeman JM, Pillas DJ, Pyzik PL. The Ketogenic Diet: A 3 to 6 year follow-up of 150 children enrolled prospectively. *Pediatrics* 2001;108:898–905.

Hong AM, Hamdy RF, Turner Z, Kossoff EH. Infantile spasms treated with the ketogenic diet: Prospective single-center experience in 104 consecutive infants. *Epilepsia*2010;51:1403–1407.

Kim DW, Kang HC, Park JC, Kim HD. Benefits of the nonfasting ketogenic diet compared with the initial fasting ketogenic diet. *Pediatrics*2004;114:1627–1630.

Kossoff EH. More fat and fewer seizures: Dietary therapy for epilepsy. *Lancet Neurol* 2004;3:415–420.

Kossoff EH, Hedderick EF, Turner Z, Freeman JM. A case-control evaluation of the ketogenic diet versus ACTH for new-onset infantile spasms. *Epilepsia*2008;49:1504–1509.

Kossoff EH, Krauss GL, McGrogan JR, Freeman JM. Efficacy of the Atkins Diet as therapy for intractable epilepsy. *Neurology*2003;61:1789–1791.

Kossoff EH, Laux LC, Blackford R, Morrison PF, Pyzik PL, Turner Z, Nordli DR, Jr. When do seizures improve with the ketogenic diet? *Epilepsia* 2008;49:329–333.

Kossoff EH, McGrogan JR. Worldwide use of the ketogenic diet. *Epilepsia* 2005;46:280–289.

Kossoff EH, Pyzik PL, McGrogan JR, Vining EPG, Freeman JM. Efficacy of the ketogenic diet for infantile spasms. *Pediatrics* 2002;109:780–783.

Kossoff EH, Rowley H, Sinha SR, Vining EPG. A prospective study of the modified Atkins diet for intractable epilepsy in adults. *Epilepsia* 2008;49:316–319.

Kossoff EH, Zupec-Kania BA, Rho JM. Ketogenic Diets: An update for child neurologists. *J Child Neurol* 2009;24:979–988.

Kossoff EH, Zupec-Kania BA, Amark PE, Ballaban-Gil KR, Bergqvist ACG, Blackford R, Buchhalter JR, Caraballo RH, Cross JH, Dahlin MG, Donner EJ, Jehle RS, Klepper J, Kim HD, Liu YMC, Nation J, Nordli, DR Jr, Pfeifer HH, Rho JM, Stafstrom CE, Thiele EA, Turner Z, Veggiotti P, Vining EPG, Wheless JW, Wirrell

EC, Charlie Foundation, and the Practice Committee of the Child Neurology Society. Optimal clinical management of children receiving the ketogenic diet: recommendations of the international ketogenic diet study group. *Epilepsia* 2009;50:304–317.

Mady MA, Kossoff EH, McGregor AL, Wheless JW, Pyzik PL, Freeman JM. The ketogenic diet: adolescents can do it, too. *Epilepsia* 2003;44:847–51.

McNally MA, Pyzik PL, Rubenstein JE, Hamdy RF, Kossoff EH. Empiric use of Oral Potassium Citrate Reduces Symptomatic Kidney Stone Incidence with the Ketogenic Diet. *Pediatrics*2009;124:e300–e304.

Neal EG, Chaffe HM, Schwartz RH, Lawson M, Edwards N, Fitzsimmons G, Whitney A, Cross JH. The ketogenic diet in the treatment of epilepsy in children: a randomised, controlled trial. *Lancet Neurol.* 2008;7:500–506.

Nordli DR, Jr., Kuroda MM, Carroll J, et. al. Experience with the ketogenic diet in infants. *Pediatrics* 2001;108:129–133.

Patel A, Pyzik PL, Turner Z, Rubensetein JE, Kossoff EH. Long-term outcomes of children treated with the ketogenic diet in the past. *Epilepsia*2010;51:1277–1282.

Pfeifer HH, Thiele EA. Low-glycemic-index treatment: a liberalized ketogenic diet for treatment of intractable epilepsy. *Neurology* 2005;65:1810–1812.

Rubenstein JE, Kossoff EH, Pyzik PL, Vining EPG, McGrogan JR, Freeman JM. Experience in the use of the ketogenic diet as early therapy. *J Child Neurol* 2005;20:31–34.

Than KD, Kossoff EH, Rubenstein JE, Pyzik PL, McGrogan JR, Vining EPG. Can you predict an immediate, complete, and sustained response to the ketogenic diet? *Epilepsia* 2005;46:580–582.

Vining EPG, Freeman JM, for the Ketogenic Diet Study Group. A multi-center study of the efficacy of the ketogenic diet. *Arch Neurol* 1998;55:1433–1437.

Wheless JW. The Ketogenic Diet: An effective medical therapy with side effects. *J Child Neurol* 2001;16:633–635.

THE MEDIUM-CHAIN TRIGLYCERIDE (MCT) DIET

Huttenlocher PR, Wilbourn AJ, Signore JM. Medium-chain triglycerides as a therapy for intractable epilepsy. *Neurology* 1971;21:1097–1103.

Sills MA, Forsyth WI, Haidukwych D. The medium-chain triglyceride diet and intractable epilepsy. *Arch Disease in Childhood* 1986:1169–1172.

Trauner, DA. Medium-chain triglyceride (MCT) diet in intractable seizure disorders. *Neurology* 1985:237–238.

OTHER BOOKS OF INTEREST

Bowden Jonny. *Living the low carb life.* Sterling, New York, 2004.

The CalorieKing Calorie, fat and carbohydrate counter 2011. Family Health Publications, Costa Mesa, CA, 2011.

Sndyer Deborah. *Keto kid.* Demos, New York, 2007.

Stafstrom C, Rho J, editors. *Epilepsy and the ketogenic diet.* Humana Press, Totowa, NJ, 2004.

Westman EC, Phinney SD, Volek JS. *The new Atkins for a new you.* Fireside, New York, 2010.

Back Cover Material

Ketogenic DIETS
Treatments for Epilepsy and Other Disorders
FIFTH EDITON

Eric H. Kossoff, MD • John M. Freeman, MD • Zahava Turner, RD • James E. Rubenstein, MD

"It will end up being the most well-read book you own and every keto home should have one. My copy went everywhere with me when Matthew was on the diet and I can't recommend it highly enough."

—**Emma Williams,** CEO/Founder, Matthew's Friends Charity, Dietary Treatments for Epilepsy, GLOBAL; Director, Matthew's Friends Clinics Ltd. for Ketogenic Dietary Therapies

"If we had had the information in this book fifteen months earlier, a vast majority of Charlie's $100,000 of medical, surgical, and drug treatment would not have been necessary, a vast majority of Charlie's seizures would not have occurred."

—**From the Foreword by Jim Abrahams,** Director, The Charlie Foundation to Help Cure Pediatric Epilepsy

One in five children with epilepsy has seizures that are resistant to medication. Even when seizures are under control, drugs may affect children's alertness and mental clarity, impairing their ability to learn and reach their full potential. Many parents are looking beyond currently available medications for a satisfying solution to seizure treatment.

The ketogenic diet is one such answer. Sometimes referred to as a "miracle diet," the ketogenic diet has helped doctors treat difficult-to-control epileptic seizures in thousands of children. Co-authored by four respected experts from Johns Hopkins, *Ketogenic Diets* continues to be the definitive guide for parents, patients, physicians, and dieticians wanting to implement this strict diet.

This Fifth Edition has been extensively updated to reflect current advances in understanding how the diet works, how it should be used, and the future role of the diet as a treatment. Six new chapters address how to integrate the diet into all cultures, religions, and taste preferences; new information on modified and less restrictive versions of the diet, and the use of diets for adults with epilepsy are included. The book also covers exciting new research that shows how the diet may work for people with other neurological illnesses. This best-seller also includes sample meal plans, a food database, how to calculate foods, and much more.

A

B

C

Q

R

S

T

U

V

W

Z

Books For ALL Kinds of Readers

At ReadHowYouWant we understand that one size does not fit all types of readers. Our innovative, patent pending technology allows us to design new formats to make reading easier and more enjoyable for you. This helps improve your speed of reading and your comprehension. Our EasyRead printed books have been optimized to improve word recognition, ease eye tracking by adjusting word and line spacing as well as minimizing hyphenation. Our EasyRead SuperLarge editions have been developed to make reading easier and more accessible for vision-impaired readers. We offer Braille and DAISY formats of our books and all popular E-Book formats.

Made in United States
North Haven, CT
05 November 2026

21767040R00293